INSPECTOR BODYGUARD™
PATROLS THE LAND OF U

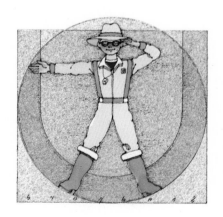

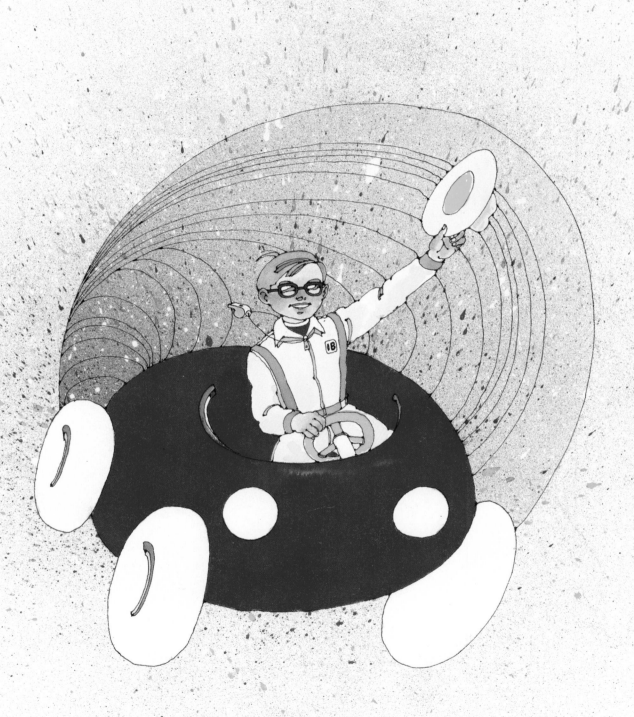

INSPECTOR BODYGUARD™
PATROLS THE LAND OF U

Vicki Cobb

Illustrated by John Sandford

Julian Messner
Published by Simon & Schuster, Inc. New York

The author and publisher thank Stephen Atwood, M.D.,
Associate Professor of Clinical Pediatrics,
Columbia-Presbyterian College of Physicians
and Surgeons, for reading the manuscript of this book.

Text Copyright © 1986 by Vicki Cobb
Illustrations Copyright © 1986 by John Sandford
Designed by Judith Murello

Manufactured in the United States of America

10 9 8 7 6 5 4 3 2 1   (lib. bdg.)

10 9 8 7 6 5 4 3 2 1   (pbk.)

Library of Congress Cataloging-in-Publication Data:

Cobb, Vicki. Inspector Bodyguard patrols the land of U.

Includes index. Summary: Inspector Bodyguard's response to a splinter in the foot and attack by cold germs intro-
duces the human body's defense system. 1. Immune response—Juvenile literature. 2. Body, Human—Juvenile liter-
ature. [1. Immunity] I. Sandford, John 1948-   ill. II. Title.
QR 181.8.C63   1986   616.07'9   86-8334
ISBN 0-671-60306-X (lib. bdg.)
ISBN 0-671-63260-4 (pbk.)

For Frank

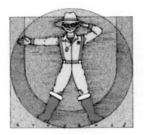

CONTENTS

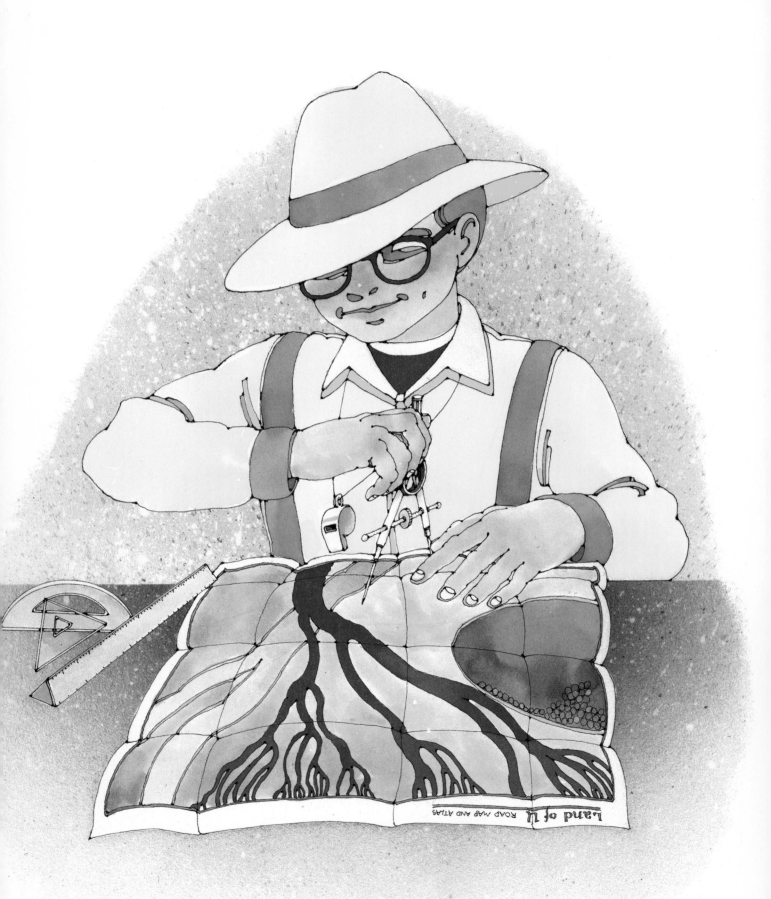

INSPECTOR BODYGUARD™
PATROLS THE LAND OF U

I am always on the go,
On the job from head to toe.
I right the wrongs that come this way
No matter what the time of day.

Who am I?

"Inspector Bodyguard" is my name
Body fitness is my game.
Come with me now
See what I do
To keep the health
In the Land of U.

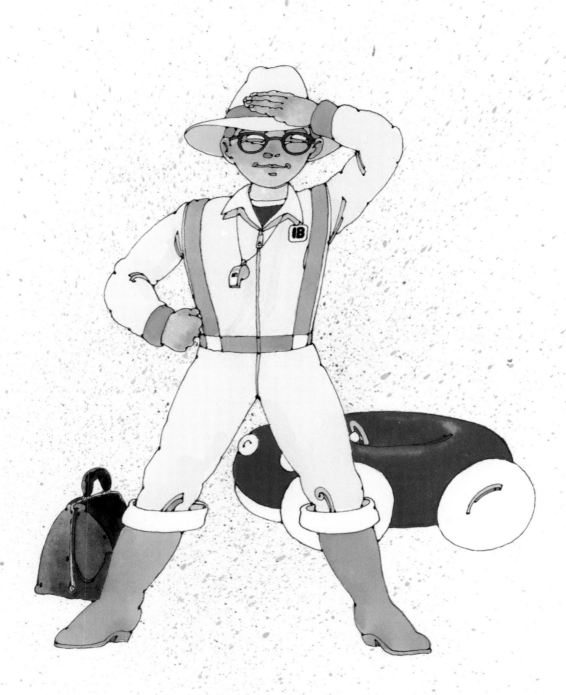

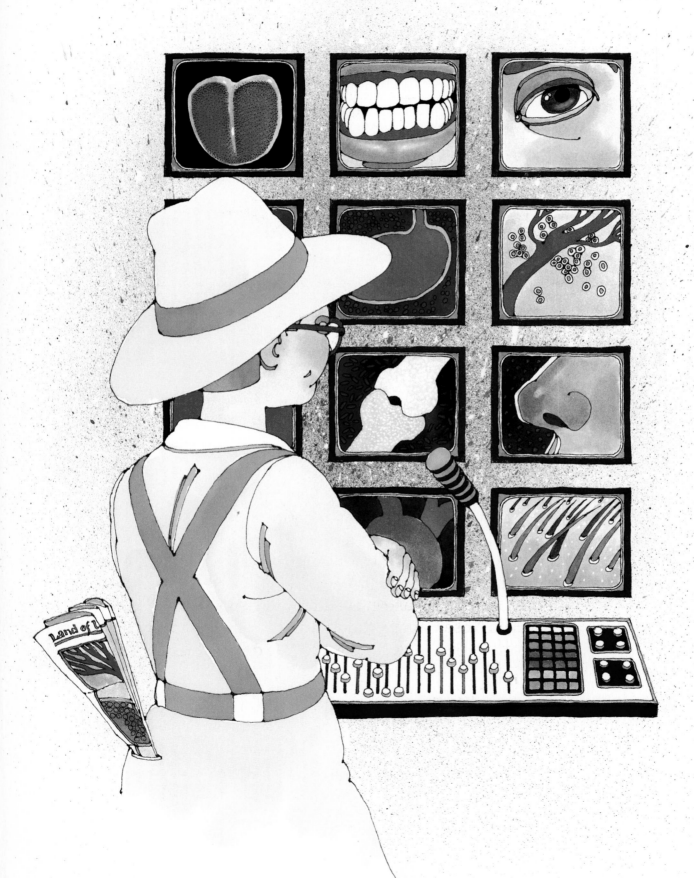

1:

THE INVASION OF SINUS HILL

On an ordinary day in the Land of U, its trillions of cell citizens are busy at work. Each has a special job to do. Red Cell Truckers make oxygen deliveries to every part of the nation, from Scaly Scalp to Toeprint Ridge. Sensing cells send messages to muscle cells through the Axon Messenger Service. Now muscle cells can pull their own weight by making the right moves at the right time. Villi cells in Small Gut Tunnel take in the daily food shipment. And on Sinus Hill, in Nose Cavern, thousands upon thousands of Living Hair Cells work together, sweeping out the dust that comes in with the air from the Great Beyond.

Inspector Bodyguard, Keeper of the Health, keeps his eye on things all over this great land from his office at Cortex Central. "What a country!" he thinks to himself. "This is what life should be. Everyone working together. Everything running smoothly. Beautiful. Simply beautiful!" For the Inspector, such peace and harmony means a slow day at the office.

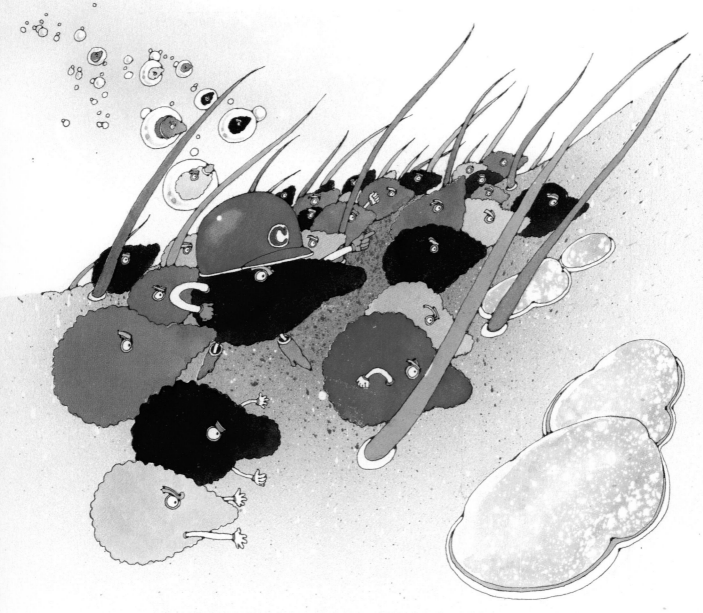

But not for long! Danger lurks in the Great Beyond. A cloud of glittering water balls drifts towards the Land of U. In each droplet is a unit of cold virus troopers. Taken all together they make up that fearsome menace—the Cold Virus Army—led by General Cold Virus himself!

General Cold Virus commands from the chief droplet at the head of the squadron. "General Cold Virus here to troops. General Cold Virus to troops. Prepare to attack. Target dead…heh! heh! …ahead. Sinus Hill in the Land of U…Get ready. The next intake of air will carry us home."

With a whoosh and a swoosh the entire Cold Virus Army is carried into Nose Cavern under its dark red, hairy ceiling.

Below, the unsuspecting cell citizens are minding their own business. Goblet cells gently send small gobs of clear, thick mucus to the surface. Millions of tiny gobs run together to make a thin film over all the cells of Sinus Hill. It keeps things clean and protected from some of the soot and other air pollution that comes in with air from the Great Beyond. The Living Hair Cells gently wave back and forth like fields of wheat. As they work they sing loud and clear:

> We do what we must
> To keep out the dust
> Yo ho heave ho!
> By waving fast
> Nothing gets past
> Yo ho heave ho!
>
> We concoct a brew
> Of slimy goo
> Yo ho heave ho!
> It traps the dust
> That sticks to us
> Yo ho heave ho!
>
> Up, up, and away
> We sweep and sweep
> Yo ho heave ho!
> When U are awake
> And when U are asleep
> Yo ho heave ho!

No one suspects the enemy above.

Then, General Cold Virus gives the dread command: "Take it down, troops!"

The almost invisible army lands on Sinus Hill. Immediately, the cold virus troops give an injection into the cell citizens. The substance of the injection uses the body of a cell citizen to begin making carbon copies of itself. The stricken cell citizens get fatter and fatter as they fill up with viruses. Cries of distress are heard all along the Hill.

"Help…help. I'm going to explode."

"I can't stand feeling this full."

"Go copy yourself someplace else. What do you need me for?"

The goblet cells do their very best as a first line of defense. They begin popping gobs faster and faster. "Let's flood them out of here!" they yell to each other. Soon Sinus Hill is like a waterfall and the connecting air passages become rivers.

Suddenly a giant disturbance, almost like an explosion, shakes the entire Land of U. It knocks Inspector Bodyguard off his stool.

"Suffering synapses! That could only be a sneezequake. I'd better get to Sinus Hill on the double."

The Inspector quickly jumps into his Blood Buggy, which is parked in a nearby bloodstream, and whips into the closest artery for a fast trip to Sinus Hill. Fortunately, Cortex Central is not far from the scene of the invasion.

"Whatever's causing the trouble," thinks Inspector Bodyguard, "I'd better alert the White Cell Civil Defense Squad, better known as the Germbusters." The Inspector activates his Sensory Alarm System. "Calling Germbusters. Calling Germbusters. Captain Blast, come in. Over."

Not far away, in Nodesville, Captain Blast hears the call.

"Captain Blast here, Inspector. I felt the sneezequake and figured you'd be calling. What do you think? Cold Virus Army or just a piece of dust that got past the Living Hair Cells?"

"Can't tell till I get there, Blast. What shape is your squad in?" asks the Inspector.

"You know how they are. Nothing very regular here until they start to move."

"Well, the Antibody Division had better tool up. We'll need a stockpile of antibodies—and fast. You know they're our ultimate weapon. That's an order, Blast."

"Right, Inspector. We'll start making antibodies as soon as we know the shape of the enemy."

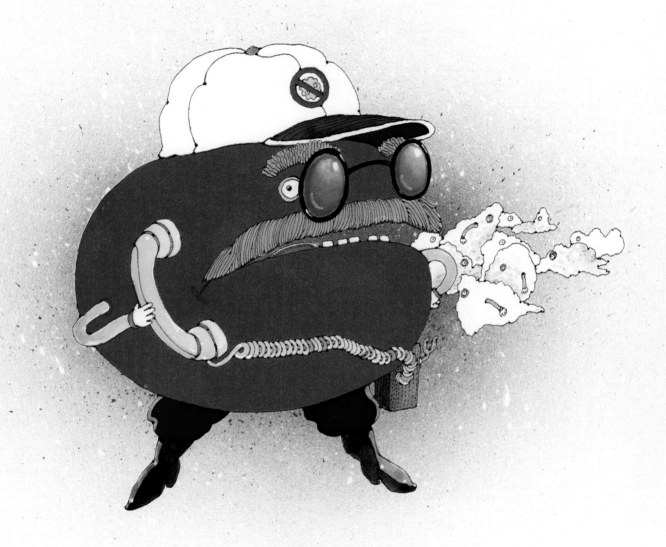

A grim sight greets the Inspector as he arrives at Sinus Hill. The living hair cells are totally flattened under the river of mucus. The air passages are completely clogged. And the goblet cells have pulled out all stops and are spilling gobs out of control. The entire Land of U is suffering.

But if the goblet cells are out of control, Inspector Bodyguard is not. As things get tougher, he gets cooler.

"Calling Captain Blast, over," says the Inspector into his Sensory Alarm System.

"Blast, here, Inspector. How does it look?"

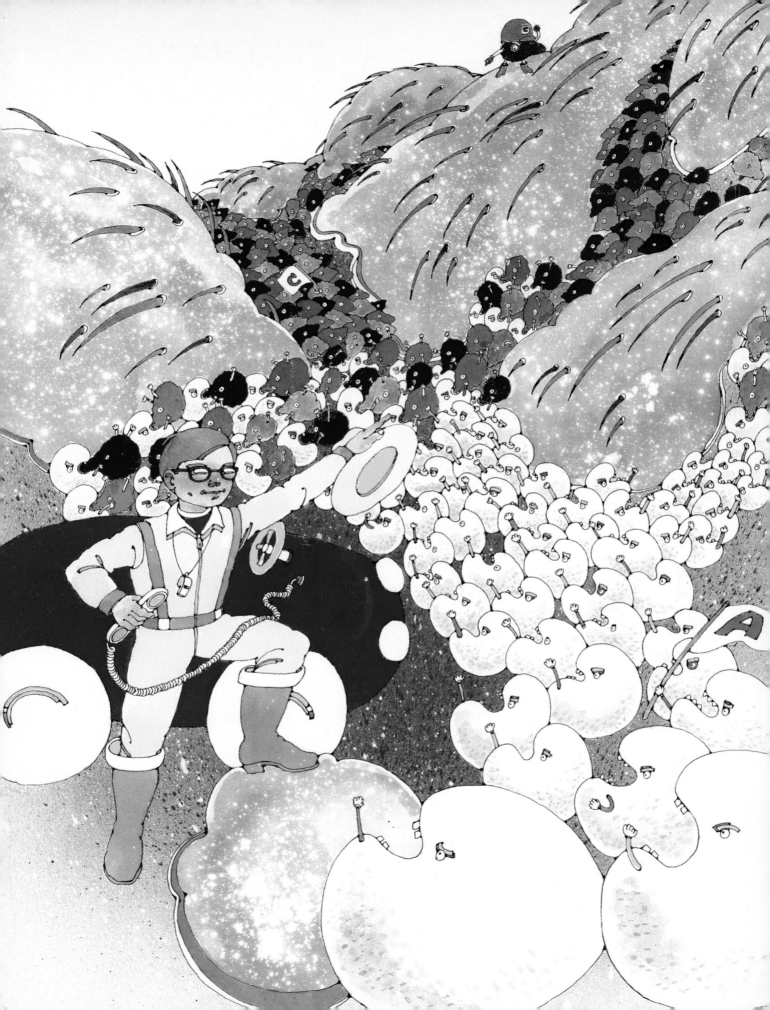

"It's those almost invisible cold viruses, Blast. A local battle that will last only three days if we get right on it."

"Roger, Inspector. We're ready to move." Captain Blast turns toward his squad. "It's the Cold Virus Army. Get out the blueprints and start antibody production A-S-A-P." To the Inspector the Captain says, "We're on top of it, sir, over."

The White Cell Ammo Factory swings into action. Great stocks of raw gamma globulin are fed into the cell machinery. Out cranks finished antibodies, custom-designed to fight the cold virus troopers, one on one.

Meanwhile, back on Sinus Hill, there is death and destruction. In some cells, cold virus troops had made so many copies of themselves that they had split law-abiding cell citizens wide open. Freshly made cold virus troops are rushing to invade other unsuspecting, untouched cell citizens.

Inspector Bodyguard paces up and down at the border between Nose Cavern and Upper Lip, jumping over streams of mucus. "Blast it, where's Blast? He'd better get here in a hurry."

Finally. the call from the good Captain, "We're ready to roll, Inspector."

"Good show, Captain. Move on in."

Loaded with antibodies, the Germbusters begin their counter-attack on the battlefield. Awesome, indeed.

"Ready…aim…fire!" yells Captain Blast.

The battle is now in earnest. Antibodies begin confronting the cold virus troopers, one by one.

"What do you think you're going to do?" asks a tough cold virus trooper of an antibody. The antibody smiles and says, "I'm going to agglutinate you!" The antibody latches onto the cold virus. A perfect fit, like two pieces of a jigsaw puzzle.

"I have a feeling we belong together," says another antibody to a cold virus. "Help! Help!" cries the virus as the antibody attaches to his front. "Now I can't copy myself."

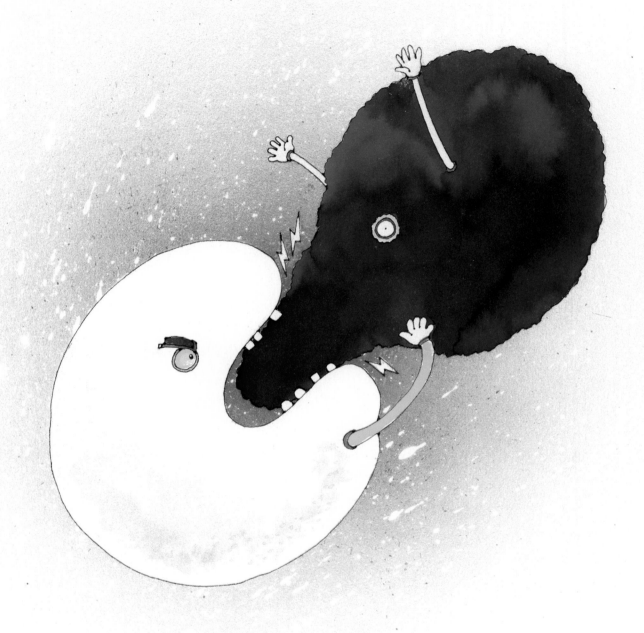

"That's the general idea," mutters the antibody.

As the antibodies take the viruses out of action, many cell citizens start recovering.

"Boy, am I glad to see you," says a Living Hair Cell to an antibody. "I can't wait to start waving again."

"I'm thirsty," says a goblet cell to no one in particular. "No wonder," thinks the Inspector, "the poor things have been working overtime. The Land of U always needs extra liquids during a cold virus invasion."

The battle rages for the usual three days. But there is never any question that the Cold Virus Army will be defeated. The flood drains off. The cell citizens return to normal size. The Living Hair Cells lift up their heads and start waving again.

Inspector Bodyguard and Captain Blast look over the scene.

"It's funny how those cold viruses never learn that they can't win," says the Inspector. "I guess they need to invade Sinus Hill in our Land of U to make copies of themselves. Then some virus troops can leave in droplets to strike some other land in the Great Beyond. That's the way they stay alive."

"Maybe someday we'll find a way to have antibodies ready for them the way we have stockpiled antibodies for polio and small-pox. We import those antibodies into the Land of U by injection," says Captain Blast.

"Well, let's hope so, Blast. Meantime, we'll just be ready for these three-day sieges. And the usual happy ending."

Inspector Bodyguard steps into his Blood Buggy to return to Cortex Central. All's well again in the Land of U.

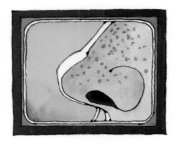

HOW
YOUR BODY FIGHTS A COLD

Every breath you take brings foreign matter into your body. Air usually contains some dust, but it also may contain germs, tiny viruses and bacteria, that can only be seen with a microscope. Normally, the foreign material that comes into your nose presents no problem. That's because the nose is set up to keep the foreign material from causing trouble.

The skin lining the nose has several different kinds of cells that act as a defense against harmful particles in the air. First there are nasal hairs that trap the really large pieces of dust. Further back are *cilia* cells, the living hair cells in the story. Many cilia line the back part of the nose and air passages and beat together, moving trapped particles toward the nostrils and out of the body. *Goblet cells*, just under the skin surface, make mucus. Under normal conditions, the goblet cells in your nose and air passages make about a quart of mucus a day. This is enough to cover the entire inside surface of skin with a thin film that keeps

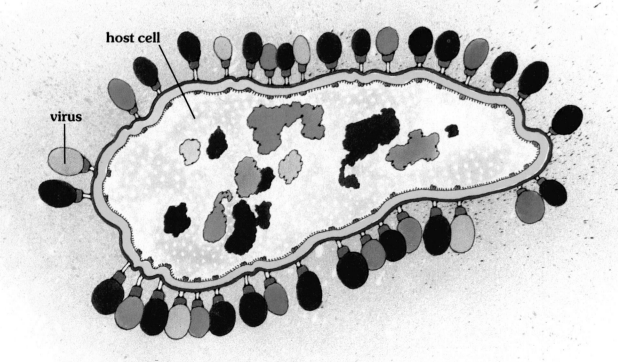

host cell

virus

foreign particles from getting into the skin. It also provides a moist, sticky surface that acts as a trap for particles and gives the cilia a chance to sweep them out.

A cold virus is extremely small, smaller than the average cell. It is hard to think of a virus as a living thing because it does not do what living things usually do unless it is on the inside of another living cell. A virus cannot take in food, give off waste, or multiply itself unless it is taking advantage of some other, more complete living cell, called the *host*. And usually, when a virus enters a host cell it causes problems for the host that show up as a disease.

The cells lining your nose and air passages are perfect hosts for cold viruses. Cold viruses get past the hairs, the cilia and the mucus, and attach themselves to the outside of the nasal skin cells. They inject their insides into the cells and take over the internal workings of the cells to make new viruses. It is like an enemy that takes over a factory and uses the factory's machinery to destroy it. When enough viruses have been made inside the cell, the cell bursts open and dies, spilling the freshly made viruses into the area so that they can infect other cells. One response to this invasion is an increase in mucus production by the goblet cells, causing a runny nose. It is an attempt by the nose to wash the viruses out of the body. But it is not enough. The invasion of a cold virus makes the body call up its second line of defense, the white blood cells.

Your blood is made up of a clear fluid called *plasma* and several kinds of cells. *Red blood cells*, which give blood its color, are red because they contain iron. (Iron metal is gray, but when iron combines with oxygen, it becomes red, like rust.) It is the job of red cells to carry oxygen from the lungs to all the other cells of the body. Red cells are extremely small. A drop of blood has about five million of them. All red cells are alike.

White blood cells make up the second group of cells in the blood. There is one white cell for about every 500 red cells. There are about six different kinds of white cells. They work together to fight germs that enter the body. Here's how.

One kind of white cell makes antibodies. To understand how antibodies work, let's backtrack a little.

All living things are built out of tiny building blocks called molecules. There are many different kinds of molecules: water, salt, carbon dioxide, and sugar are all made of molecules. The most important molecules that make up living things are proteins. A protein molecule is huge compared to a water or salt molecule. And protein molecules are very complicated. There are countless kinds of protein molecules. One way scientists tell the difference between protein molecules is by their shape. A particular protein, a protein in a cold virus, for example, has a shape that no other kind of protein has. An antibody for this virus must be custom-made so that its shape fits exactly into the shape of the virus protein, like a key in a lock.

Lymphocytes, a kind of white blood cell, manufacture antibodies to fit cold viruses out of a protein called globulin. (Gamma globulin is a particular kind of globulin.) These antibodies have the *exact opposite* shape of a part of the virus protein. When an antibody meets a germ, they lock together. The virus can then no longer invade host cells. This process of locking together is called *agglutination*. If you saw agglutination in a test tube, you would see a clear solution become cloudy as the antibodies and germs join.

There are other white cells called *monocytes* and *macrophages*, which travel to the sight of infection. Monocytes have no regular shape. They move by changing their shape. One side of a cell begins to stick out like a knob and the rest of the cell pours itself into the knob. This kind of moving is called *ameboid motion*, named after the *ameba*, a one-celled animal that also travels this way.

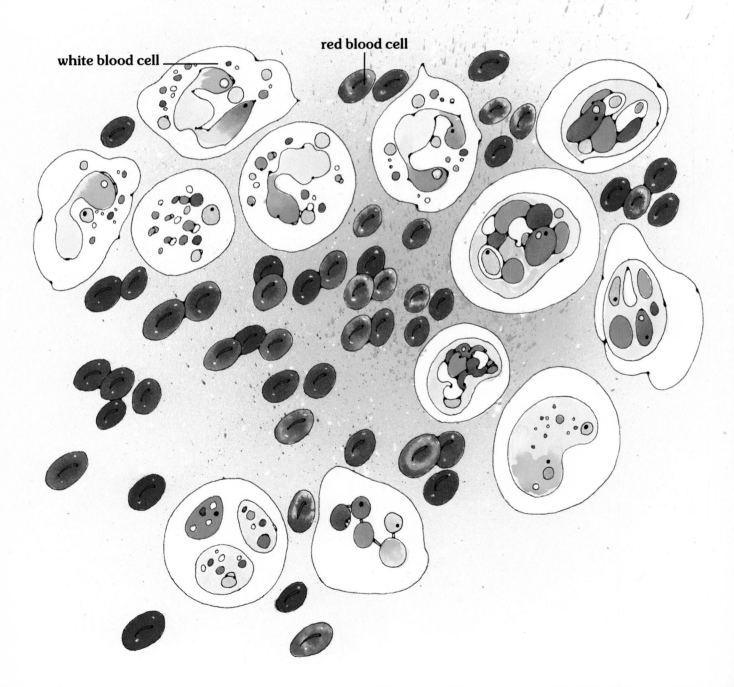

Amebas can be found by looking at a drop of water from a pond under a microscope. White cells with ameboid motion can squeeze themselves through tiny spaces between cells that make up the walls of blood vessels. They move freely to the area that needs them most. Monocytes and macrophages kill germs by "eating" them. The next story will tell you more about macrophages that "hunger" after bacteria.

There is another fluid in your body besides blood that travels to all your cells. It is called *lymph*. Like blood, lymph moves between cells, it also collects in tubular vessels that come together in various places around your body. Lymph vessels meet in *lymph nodes*. There are lymph nodes in your neck and under your arm, for example. A few of the germs at the site of an infection will get picked up by the lymph and wind up at a lymph node. There, the lymph is filtered and all the dead white cells are removed. Sometimes, when you are sick and your lymph nodes are working overtime, they get swollen. This condition is often called "swollen glands," although your lymph nodes are not really glands.

After a cold, the white cells clear away all traces of the battle, the swelling goes down, and the cells of the nose lining multiply and replace the ones destroyed by the infection.

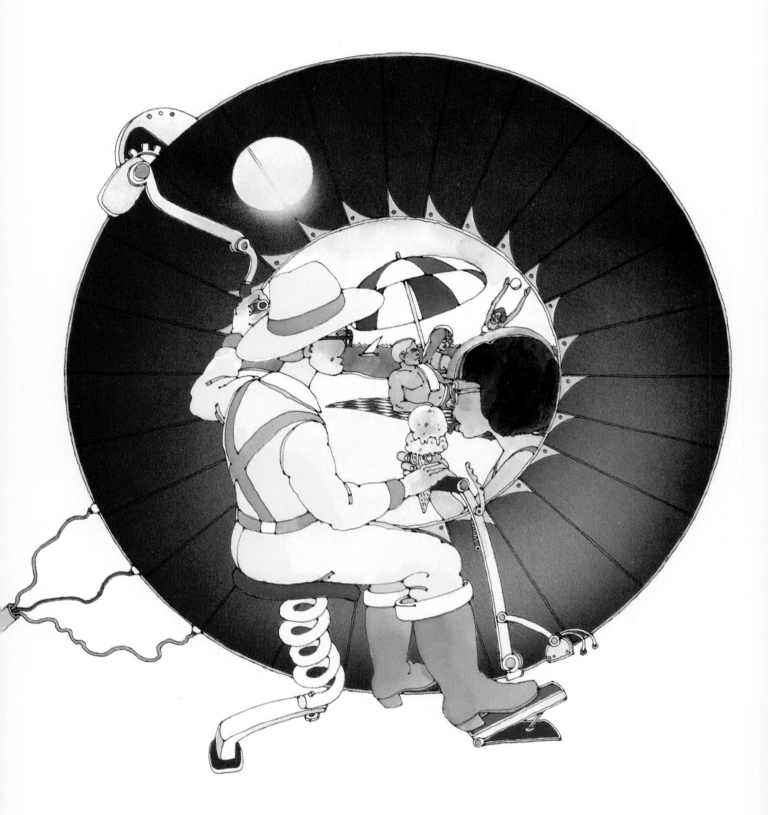

2:

THE SIEGE ON TOEPRINT RIDGE

It is a hot, blue summer day in the Great Beyond. The Land of U is at the beach. Inspector Bodyguard is enjoying himself as he watches the sights of the Great Beyond from his favorite observation point in Pupil Park. "Hmmm. That Human Body is going to create problems for her inspector with that sunburn," he comments to himself as Pupil Park turns toward a red sunbather. "And that young Human Body is putting his Belly Bag through a difficult time. Not good…processing all that junk food at one time."

The Inspector presses his lips together and shakes his head. "A day at the beach can create problems for me, too. I know that Toeprint Ridge is taking an extra beating today…no shoes and all that hot sand. I think I'll go give some moral support to the Skin Cell citizens down there."

The Inspector turns away from the round window of Pupil Park and moves through the clear jellylike Vitreous Pond to Retina Image Dish at its shore. Retina Image Dish is full of small blood vessels that connect with the Land of U's incredible Arterial Network that can take the Inspector to any part of the Land he wishes to visit. The Inspector gets into his Blood Buggy and consults his map. "Let's see…Hmmm. If I make the correct turns I should be at Toeprint Ridge, at the other end of the Land of U, in about five minutes." The Inspector settles back for a relaxed journey.

He doesn't notice that the Land of U has turned and is moving toward the wooden boardwalk.

Inspector Bodyguard knows he is near the end of his journey when he hears the chorus of Skin Cells singing their mournful "Lament."

> As tender young cells
> we're born far from the surface,
> with layers of cells between us and
>   the ground.
> Then new cells behind us
> push us toward the front lines.
> We toughen inside
> as for death we are bound.
>
> You can see by our toughness
> that we are old Skin Cells
> whose job is to keep out the germs
>   that fly by.
> Our dead bodies give U
> front-line protection.
> It's our honor and duty
> to lie down and die.

The Inspector moves among the Skins Cells at the Granular Layer, those just about to die. "I want to thank you all for doing a fine job for the greater good of the Land of U."

"It's our pleasure, Inspector," says an old, grainy cell. "After all, it's the reason we were born twenty-seven days ago. We are about to become the Land of U's personal shoe leather."

"Our whole life is about getting tougher and tougher," adds a

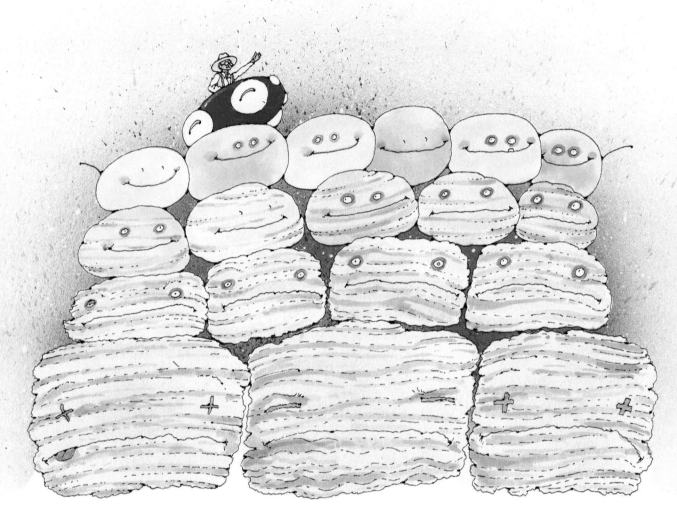

slightly younger Prickle Cell. "But we're toughest of all after we die. And we're proud of it!"

The Inspector is just about to congratulate the Skin Cells on their positive attitude when suddenly a giant, dark brown, spearlike object is thrust roughly into their midst.

The Skin Cells in the path of the object are fatally wounded. Their cries can be heard by the surrounding cells.

"Help, help! I'm too young to die," cries a youthful Basal Skin Cell.

"Oh dear. We can't protect against a nasty splinter. I've seen this kind of thing before," says an old, grainy cell.

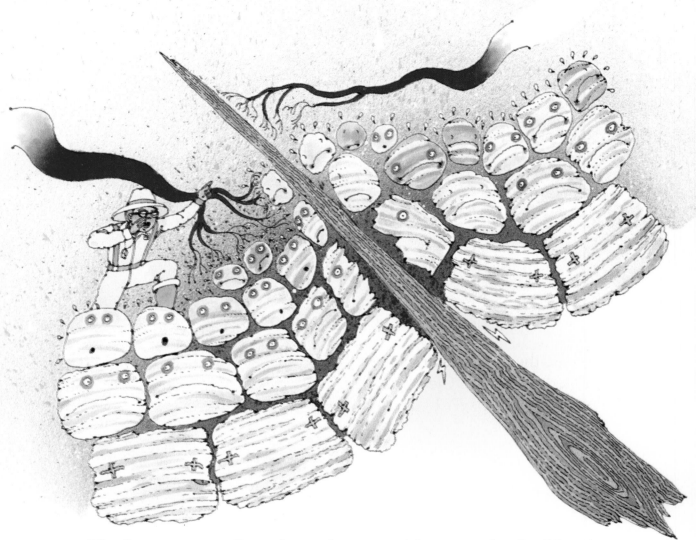

The Inspector is yelling above the cries of the injured cells. "Send out your liquid warning! Send out your liquid warning! We've got to start the Inflammation Defense Reaction immediately!"

The Inspector watches for a few moments while the injured cells give a last gasp and squirt the surrounding cells with a warning splash. When the warning hits a small blood vessel there is an instant reaction. It quickly expands, letting gushes of blood rush into the area.

The Inspector smiles with satisfaction. "That will warm things up for the germs on the splinter. I'd better get Captain Blast here." The Inspector turns on his handy Sensory Alarm System. "Captain Blast, come in, please. Emergency. Over."

"Blast here, Inspector," comes the soothing voice of the head of the White Cell Civil Defense Squad, better known as the Germbusters. "What's the problem, sir?"

"We've got a dirty splinter puncture on Toeprint Ridge, Blast. The warning splash has produced the usual rush of blood, but the next step is up to you."

"Right, Inspector. I'm mobilizing the Big Macro Germ Eating Unit to start cleaning up the debris. Better open the blood serum valves. We want to put pressure on the area. Too bad, but Land of U has got to feel some pain. I'm on my way to the site of siege."

True to Captain Blast's word, the Big Macros start squeezing themselves into the area. They begin sending armlike lobes of their shapeless bodies around either side of the germs. When they come together at the other side of an enemy, they blend together and bingo!—the germ is inside the Macro. Fearsome, indeed! In this way the Macros start cleaning up the mess caused by the splinter's puncture. Clear, yellowish fluid begins seeping around the splinter. The cells begin to feel pressed by the swelling.

"I can't understand it," mutters the Inspector to himself. "Why hasn't the Land of U pulled out the splinter?"

The Inspector turns to a nearby Deep Pressure Nerve Cell. "Aren't you sending a pain message to Brain Command Post?"

"Yes sir, Inspector, at eighty miles an hour."

"So why hasn't Brain made the Land of U remove the splinter. Doesn't Brain feel pain?"

"I think, sir," Deep Pressure Nerve says slowly, "that Brain is too busy with the fun of the beach. Brain is ignoring our message."

"Brain has some nerve! Imagine ignoring an important message of pain! Now the germs on the splinter will really make themselves at home. Did you hear what's happening, Blast?"

Captain Blast has come up beside the Inspector. "We'll just have to keep up the pressure. But it's going to be worse than it need be." The Captain shakes his head sadly as he watches an eager

Big Macro eat its fifteenth germ. It proves to be that Big Macro's last germ; it dies of overeating shortly thereafter.

"I'm glad Big Macros have the stomach for this necessary but unpleasant job," comments the Inspector.

"They're just doing what they're made for. They have a built-in appetite for germs. To them, germ-eating is gourmet dining," says Captain Blast.

Meanwhile, the germ enemies that entered with the invading splinter are as happy as pigs in mud.

"Great gobs of goo! This place is sure wet and warm. A perfect place to grow fat!" One rod-shaped germ begins guzzling fluids.

"No air. No sun. This is my kind of place! I'm fat enough now to split in two. In fact, that's just what I'll do." The germ suddenly divides into two smaller versions of itself. Each one begins eating as if its life depends on it.

"Cornified corns!" exclaims the Inspector. "Did you see that, Blast. We're going to be overrun! They're disgusting! Look at them sitting in their own wastes!"

"Very irritating," agrees Captain Blast.

Suddenly, after much crying by the Skin Cells and strong pain messages from the Nerve Cells, the splinter is removed, taking thousands of germs with it. Needless to say, no one is sorry to see them go.

"Whew!" says the Inspector. "That makes our job a lot easier." He turns toward the battlefield. "Brace yourselves for the hydrogen peroxide flood."

The Nerve Cells concentrate. This is an unpleasant message they have to send to Brain Command Post. Hydrogen peroxide flood makes a slight sting. BCP does not especially want to receive it. But it could be worse. Iodine on the wound really hurts.

Hydrogen peroxide washes into the area. Soon bubbles of oxygen are released by a substance in the blood. Germs can be heard complaining all over.

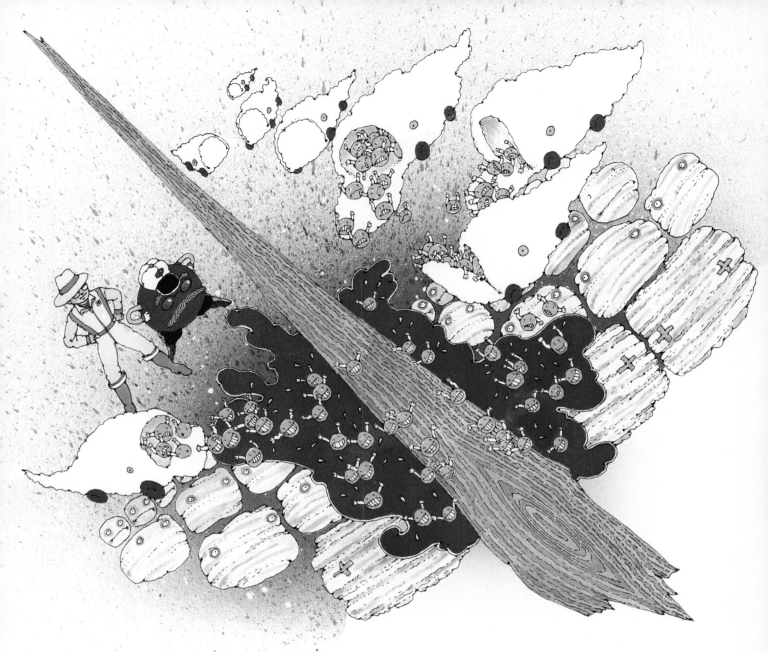

"Where did that stuff come from? Gas warfare isn't fair!"

"Oxygen stunts my growth."

"Oh well, it was nice here while it lasted."

"What do you think, Inspector?" asks Captain Blast. "How long will this siege last?"

"Well, if the splinter had stayed in, it would have been a long and painful battle. But now we've turned the corner. A few more days and the blood vessels can shrink to normal. And the deepest layer of Skin Cells can start replacing itself. In my opinion, Blast, this is just a minor skirmish."

HOW YOUR BODY FIGHTS INFECTION

The inside of your body is ideal for the nourishment and growth of many kinds of bacteria, tiny one-celled plants that are found everywhere on earth. Some bacteria do especially well in the warm, moist, oxygen-free environment provided by the tissues of your body. So the first line of defense against such germs is your skin.

Your skin is a waterproof bag with an irregular shape. When you are grown, it will cover about two square yards and will weigh about fourteen pounds. In addition to keeping out bacteria, the skin does several other important jobs. It gets rid of waste through sweat glands. It helps keep you warm when it's cold and cools you off when it's warm. It protects you from harmful sun rays. And it keeps you from drying out. It is built to protect you from the wear and tear of contact with the world. The skin at the bottoms of your feet is especially good at this job. It is the toughest skin of your body.

It is also the thickest. Like all your skin, the skin at the bottoms of your feet has two layers, the *epidermis* and the *dermis*. The epidermis is the outer layer and is the scene of the story. There are five layers of cells in the epidermis. The deepest layer is made of *basal* skin cells. Basal cells are rapidly dividing in two all the time, providing new skin cells. As these cells are pushed toward the surface, they become many-sided, making them look prickly. Such "prickly cells" contain the pigment grains that give skin its color. As these cells move closer to the surface, they lose their pigment grains and start getting grains of a tough protein called *keratin*.

As the grainy keratin cells move toward the surface, they die and become a twenty-five-to-thirty-cell layer of flat dead cells called the *stratum corneum*, meaning "cornified layer." These dead cells act as scales and are continually worn away as the skin rubs against other surfaces. The feet have a fifth, extremely tough, clear layer that is almost pure keratin. This fifth layer only appears where there is a great deal of wear and tear and often makes up those annoying pressure point on toes called "corns."

The living cells of the epidermis are nourished by blood vessels in the underlying dermis. The dermis also contains sweat glands, special bodies for detecting heat, cold, and pressure, and free nerve endings that detect pain. There are no hairs on the bottoms of the feet.

An injury, such as a splinter, that penetrates the skin, sets off a series of events. Injured cells in the path of the splinter give off a chemical called *histamine*. When histamine lands on a blood vessel, the blood vessel immediately expands, allowing more blood to rush to the area. The area surrounding the wound becomes red, warm, and painful. (The release of histamine also causes rashes and hives. If you have an allergic reaction that produces hives, a doctor will often give you an *antihistamine*, which produces the opposite effect of histamine.)

As the blood vessels expand, a clear liquid from the blood oozes into the wound area through spaces between the cells that make up the walls of blood vessels. This is blood serum. This increase in the fluid around a wound causes local swelling. Swelling walls off the infection and keeps it local.

Also squeezing through the walls of the expanded blood vessels are the amebalike *macrophages* (pronounced mac-row-fah-jes). Macrophages are huge white blood cells that engulf foreign objects that penetrate the skin. They kill germs by "eating" them. Two knobs grow out of the side of the macrophage around each side of the germ. When the two knobs meet, they join together, surrounding the germ, and suddenly the germ is inside the cell. Powerful juices then digest the germ.

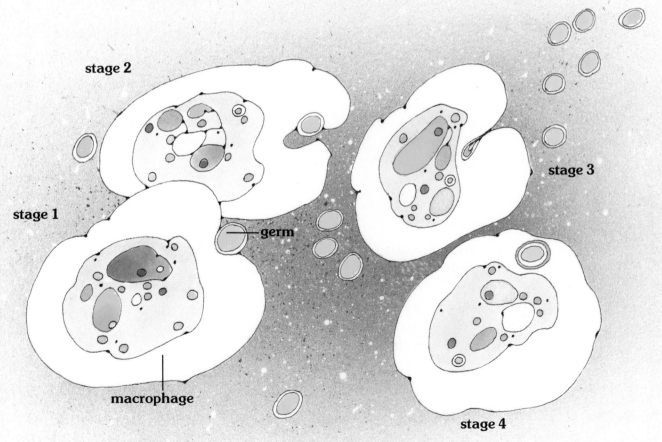

stage 2

stage 3

stage 1

germ

macrophage

stage 4

The bacteria that enter the epidermis on the surface of a splinter begin multiplying rapidly. A single bacterium splits in two every twenty minutes. In the process it gives off irritating and sometimes very harmful waste products. In the battle between the macrophages and the germs, the macrophages can "eat" just so many germs before they themselves die. Dead white cells show up as *pus* in infections and as thick white and green mucus when you blow your nose at the end of a cold. Such pus often means that the infection is almost over.

How serious an infection becomes depends mainly on how many bacteria get a chance to feed and reproduce. The inflammation reaction can easily take care of a few invading bacteria. By removing a dirty splinter, you limit the bacteria that remain in the wound. Hydrogen peroxide floods the area with oxygen, which helps limit the growth of some bacteria.

A splinter left in the skin can cause a large, painful infection that takes a lot longer to heal.

3:

TRAFFIC JAM AT PYLORIC JUNCTION

Inspector Bodyguard is sitting with his feet up in his office in Cortex Central. He has learned from Brain Command Post that the Land of U is going to the circus. So it will be a relaxed day for all the cell citizens. Everyone benefits from a day of fun. The Inspector figures he can also take it easy. Or so he thinks.

His daydreaming is interrupted by a beep from the Axon Messenger Service on his desk. The Inspector picks up the phone, knowing it is a routine call, no emergency.

"Howya doing, Inspector? It's Papilla Taste Bud down here at Tongue Receiving Station."

"Good to hear from you, Papilla. Everything okay?"

"Everything's great, Inspector. That's why I'm calling. We're having a party down here and all of us taste buds are pretty happy. We thought we'd ask you to join the fun."

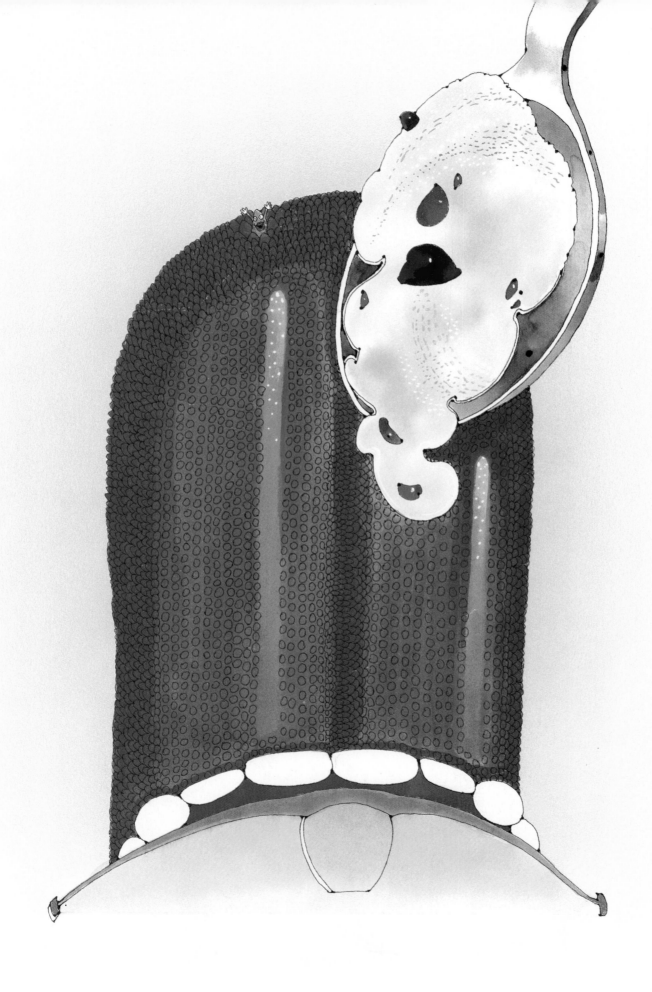

"I'm on my way, Papilla. I could use a party."

The Inspector can hear the noisy singing of the taste buds as he draws near Tongue Receiving Station. The party is in full swing!

> Happiness is here at last
> Rich, creamy goo is sloshing past
> "More, more sweet stuff!" is all we ask
> It travels by us much too fast.
>
> And now we get a salty crunch
> What better thing to have for lunch
> Than roasted peanuts by the bunch?
> Love that good stuff that U munch.
>
> Here comes a hotdog full of spice
> Who wants a dish of boiled rice?
> Glorious junk food is our vice
> It always makes us feel so nice.
>
> For it would be a shame to waste
> Yummy food U love to eat in haste.
> Our best fun is the fast food race
> Over us, the buds who sense the taste.

"Over here, Inspector," calls Papilla Taste Bud at the tip of the tongue. Papilla has a silly grin on his face. "What an experience this is. First we had cotton candy melt over us. Then we had a vanilla ice cream bath. Then we had a peanut brittle massage. Then we had a hotdog dance. Stay with us, Inspector. Enjoy it with us, whatever we get next."

The Inspector loves to see his cell citizens happy, doing what they are meant to do. He stands with Papilla at the tip of the tongue when they are suddenly thrust into the Great Beyond.

"Great sweetness and salt," cries Papilla happily. "We're getting French fries. And with ketchup!" He gazes rapturously up at the food as they move back inside Mouth Terminal.

"Don't you think you've had enough?" asks the Inspector. "A lot more has gone by than usual."

"Don't be such a sour grape, Inspector. That remark is in bad taste! We haven't had this much fun in ages. Look! Now we're getting my favorite! Chocolate candy!"

The Inspector begins to worry. Mouth Terminal and Tongue Receiving Station can handle all that food. But it is all moving too fast toward Belly Bag Waiting Room. Papilla is delirious with joy. He is certainly feeling no pain. But Inspector Bodyguard can't be sure of the rest of the Food Transport System. Mouth Terminal is just the beginning. Food from the Great Beyond still has a long journey through the Land of U. Overloading the Food Transport System can mean trouble ahead. The Inspector hears an ominous rumbling in the distance.

"Look what's coming now, Inspector. Have some with me. It's pickles and sauerkraut. Plunge right into the briny deep!"

I'd better check the Waiting Room, the Inspector thinks to himself. He quickly moves to the back of Mouth Terminal where Tongue Receiving Station has shaped some food into a ball. The Inspector hops onto the food ball and rides it down Throat Elevator to Belly Bag Waiting Room. As he fears, the waiting room is jammed.

"Who's responsible for this mess?" mutters the Inspector. He heads for a nearby nerve ending in the Belly Bag wall. "Axon Messenger Service? Get me Commander Appestat at the Appetite Control Center." His call is quickly put through to the Commander's office.

"Commander Appestat, have you gone bananas?" The Inspector's voice is intense over the wire. "You're supposed to regulate how much food comes in from the Great Beyond, keep things within limits. Can't you put a stop to any more receiving in Mouth Terminal?"

"I was expecting your call, Inspector," says Commander Appestat in a troubled tone. "I hate to say it, but I've lost control. Brain Command Post has taken over and you know that it's almost impossible to overrule Brain once he makes up his mind. I think all that junk food is going to Brain's head. The only thing we can do is teach Brain a lesson for the future."

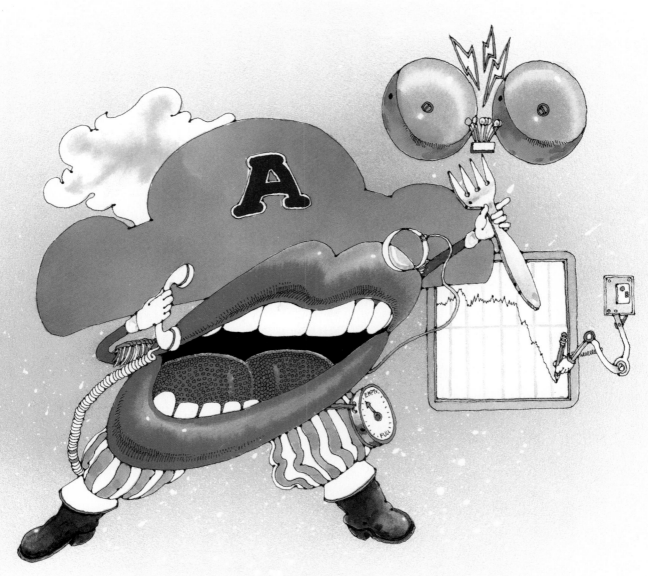

"How do you want to do that? We can empty the Waiting Room by running Throat Elevator backwards," suggests the Inspector.

"That's pretty drastic. You know how Throat Elevator hates running in reverse. What's going on at the other end of the Waiting Room, at Pyloric Junction? Maybe you can take care of it at that end," says Commander Appestat.

"I'll give it a shot. If it doesn't work, we can still pull the elevator reverse routine. Thanks for your help. Over."

Pyloric Junction is a strong exit door at the far end of Belly Bag Waiting Room. It lets food slowly out of Belly Bag into Small Gut Tunnel. On the Small Gut Tunnel side of Pyloric Junction the food is doused with strong blasts of juice from the Liver and Pancreas Chemical plants. This processes the food to be taken in and used by all the cell citizens in the Land of U. But the beginning of Small Gut Tunnel can handle just so much food at a time. Pyloric Junction has closed down under pressure. The thirty-five million cell citizens lining Belly Bag are complaining.

"Hey, Inspector. How're we supposed to handle all this stuff?"

"What's going on in Mouth Terminal, anyway? Don't they know we're stretched to the limit?"

The muscle cells in the wall of Belly Bag cry out, "How can we keep all this stuff mixed. It's too much to move!"

A pressure body in the wall tells the Inspector, "We're going to have to send pain signals to Brain. That's the only way to make him stop giving in to the taste buds."

Inspector Bodyguard throws up his hands. "Okay. Okay. Don't bellyache to me. Send the message where it counts. Meantime, I'll see what I can do to break up the traffic jam at Pyloric Junction and get that stuff moving out of here."

The Inspector wades through the backed-up food until he reaches Pyloric Junction, where he squeezes through to the other side. The walls at the beginning of Small Gut Tunnel are twisting and writhing, trying to move along a small portion of the food that has left the Waiting Room.

The Inspector gives a hard blast on his whistle.

"Citizens of Small Gut Tunnel," says the Inspector in his official Keeper of the Health voice. "May I have your attention, please. We must work together to move food out of this area as rapidly as possible and relieve the traffic jam on the other side of Pyloric Junction. Are you with me?"

The citizens of Small Gut Tunnel rumble their answer. "We're with you, Inspector."

"Okay. Pyloric Junction, give us a shot of Belly Bag contents." Pyloric Junction opens up a little, just enough to let the now liquid mixture from Belly enter Small Gut Tunnel.

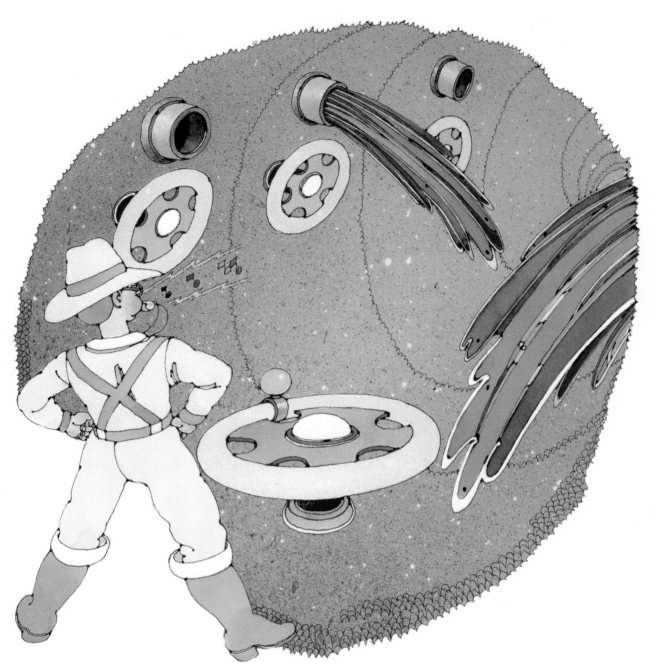

"Get ready for a shipment from the Liver and Pancreas Chemical plants. Open the valves from the Common Bile Duct." A dark brown mixture enters the Tunnel. It contains bile detergent from the liver that breaks up the fats. It also contains juice from the pancreas that processes proteins, carbohydrates and fats. It is the most powerful juice in the entire Food Transport System. Within minutes the Small Gut Tunnel is ready for more from the Waiting Room.

The Inspector stands in Small Gut Tunnel and directs traffic for two solid hours. He knows that the Land of U suffers pain from the Belly Bag Waiting Room until the pressure is relieved. On his way back to Cortex Central he stops in to see Commander Appestat.

"Well, the problem is solved, Commander. I don't think the taste buds will party quite so hard in the future. You'll be able to do your job."

"Yep, Inspector, Brain Command Post takes full responsibility for the incident. In the future, Brain will tell taste buds what to do, not the other way around."

"As it should be, Commander. All's well again in the Land of U."

The Inspector doesn't hear the taste buds whisper to each other, "Yes, but it was fun while it lasted."

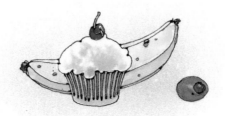

HOW
OVEREATING CAN CAUSE A BELLYACHE

All living things are made up of large, very complicated molecules. These molecules are arranged in delicate, highly organized structures. Living requires that this delicate, complex organization be maintained and for this every living thing needs food. Food is raw material used to replace worn out parts of our body and for new growth. Food also is the fuel we need for moving and growing and maintaining the high organization of our molecules that is life. (Death can be thought of as the moment when this high level of organization can no longer be maintained.)

We eat other things that were once alive. So our food is also made up of large, complicated molecules. Food molecules are slightly different from ours. But these large molecules can be broken down into simpler molecules that our bodies can use for its own purposes. This process of breaking food down is called *digestion*.

Digestion starts in the mouth. Here food is mechanically broken up by chewing and is thoroughly moistened by saliva. The chewing and wetting releases the flavor in the food. This flavor is detected by the tastebuds *papillae* and by special nerve cells in the nose. Food is supposed to taste good. If food had no taste people wouldn't enjoy eating and they might not take in the food they need to live. The pleasure of good tasting food is experienced in the brain. In fact, our appetite is also controlled by a part of the brain called the *hypothalamus*. The appetite controller in the hypothalamus is called the *appestat*. The appestat tells us when to eat and how much to eat.

The tongue shapes wet, chewed food into small balls at the back of the mouth, where it is swallowed. Swallowing moves the ball of food from the mouth to the stomach through a tube called the *esophagus*. The esophagus is a muscular tube. Rings of muscles contract, one after the other, just above the ball of food, pushing it along. This kind of motion moves food through the entire digestive system. It also lets us swallow food standing on our heads. Astronauts don't need gravity to help them eat in a weightless orbit.

The stomach is a large, j-shaped, muscular bag that stores freshly eaten food for two to six hours. The walls of the stomach move, mixing the contents, now called *chyme*, and further breaking down the food. But the main way food is now broken down is not by mechanically tearing it apart, but by chemical

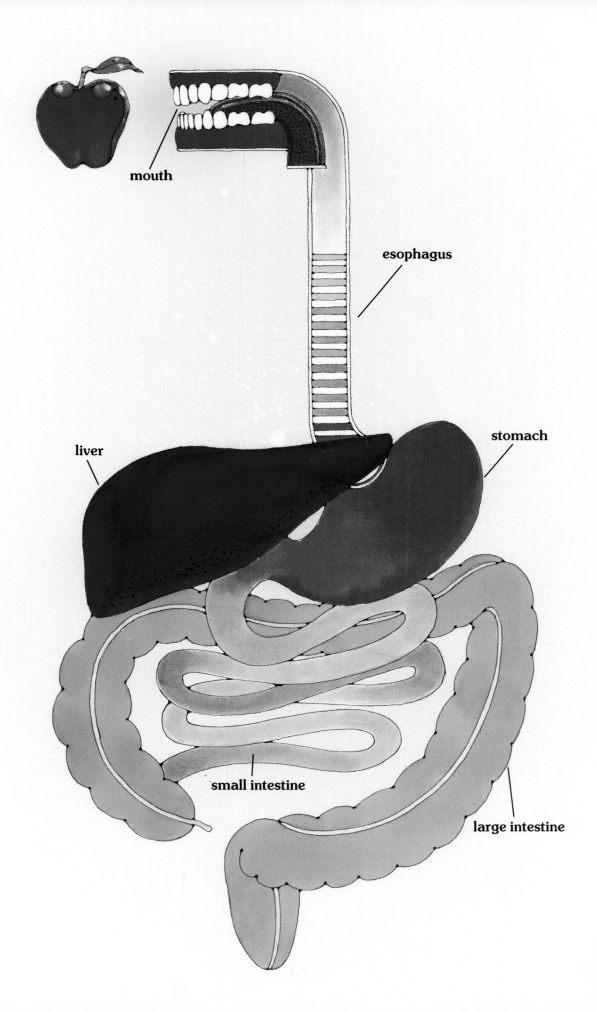

mouth

esophagus

liver

stomach

small intestine

large intestine

action. The digestive system manufactures specialized chemicals called *enzymes*. Enzymes are proteins that speed up the rate at which the chemical reactions take place. There is a different enzyme for each kind of reaction. Saliva has an enzyme that starts breaking down starches into sugars. The stomach has an enzyme that starts breaking down proteins into smaller molecules called amino acids.

Chyme is kept in the stomach by two ring-shaped muscles, called sphincters, that open and close. One sphincter is at the end of the esophagus. The other one, called the *pyloric sphincter*, is at the connection between the stomach and the small intestine. The pyloric sphincter opens and lets small amounts of chyme enter the small intestine.

Most of the chemical breakdown of food occurs in the first eight inches of the small intestine. Chyme gets zapped with *bile* from the liver and with *pancreatic juice* from the pancreas. Bile breaks up fats much as soap cuts through grease. Pancreatic juice contains enzymes that finish up carbohydrate and protein digestion and also break down fats. Now the food can be absorbed into the bloodstream as it is moved along the rest of the small intestine.

Overeating stretches the stomach walls and puts pressure on the pyloric sphincter. A lot of air is swallowed when you eat fast and gas in the stomach also presses on the stomach walls. Nerves in the stomach walls interpret this pressure as pain and send a message of pain to the brain. In time, as the chyme slowly passes out of the stomach, this pressure is relieved.

So if you get a bellyache from overeating, you can be fairly certain that it will go away within a couple of hours.

4:

FEAR TO THE RESCUE

The Land of U is playing ball with several other nations of the Great Beyond. Such activity keeps many groups of cell citizens on their toes. Muscle cells of Arm and Leg extremities are pulling together. They are using extra shipments of oxygen from the Red Cell Truckers. As a result, heart muscle cells are working harder to pump the blood to all cell citizens and the lungs are moving faster to bring in more air from the Great Beyond. Sweat glands all over Skin Frontier are pouring out liquid, helping the Land of U get rid of waste and acting as a cooling system for the extra heat generated by the intense activity.

Inspector Bodyguard is doing his job as Keeper of the Health. He keeps an eye on all his monitors from his office at Cortex Central. "So far so good," he says to himself as he goes down his checklist. "Lung Importing Company, okay. Arterial Network, Cardiac Pumping, okay. ATP Energy Delivery Stores staying well supplied. Lactic acid sludge buildup is being moved right out. No exhaustion in sight. All systems go! As it should be."

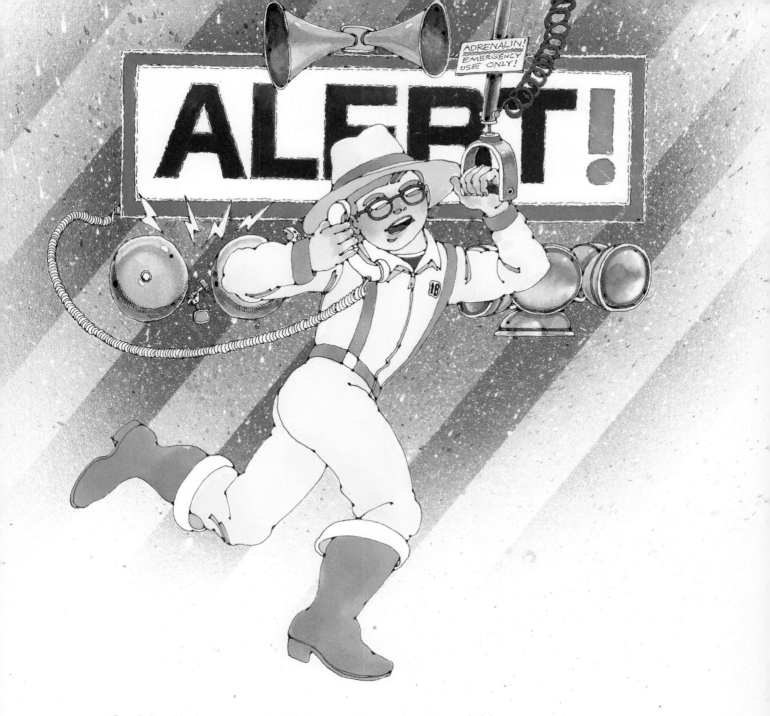

Suddenly there is a loud sound from the Great Beyond. Inspector Bodyguard instantly recognizes it as the sound of a car horn. Sirens go off in Cortex Central.

"Suffering Synapses! It's the Emergency Response Alarm setting off Startle Reflex Readiness. No time to think. I've got to prepare the Land of U for danger. Adrenalin, we need adrenalin!"

"The Inspector plugs into the Axon Messenger Service.

"Adrenal Medulla—and fast!"

A chorus of voices answers, "Secretion Service at your service, sir!"

The round cell citizens of Adrenal Medulla are standing by ready to answer the alarm.

"It's the emergency response, guys. The hot wire system has already performed Startle Reflex Readiness but we need to get set for danger. So ready…aim…squeeze adrenalin into the bloodstream."

Like fire engines to the rescue, molecules of adrenaline move into nearby blood vessels on their way to activating the Sympathetic Nervous System, a division that automatically puts the entire Land of U into a state of emergency.

"Ah…like a shot in the arm," observes the Inspector. "Now to alert the Sympathetic Nerves that the stimulant is on its way."

The Inspector commands into the wire, "Autonomic Nervous System, Sympathetic Division, come in Ganglia."

The high-strung Ganglia come on the wire. "Listen, gang," says the Inspector, "adrenalin is on its way. Prepare to transmit messages to all parts of the body."

While the Inspector is tuned in he can hear the gang of Ganglia being zapped by adrenalin molecules. Instantly the nerves respond by sending messages.

"Whew!" Inspector Bodyguard wipes his brow in relief. "Fear has been instilled in the Land of U." He glances at his watch. "Not bad timing. Less than half a second since the car horn. The wheels here are in motion. Fear Chain Reaction has begun."

Fear is not a pleasant condition for the Land of U. But in its own way it protects the great nation.

"By now the Land of U should know what the problem is. Oh, I see. It's the old-ball-in-the-street bit. I hope the Inspector of the Human Body in that car has his state of emergency in place, too."

The Inspector now turns his attention to the monitors to watch the result of the Sympathetic Nerves' messages.

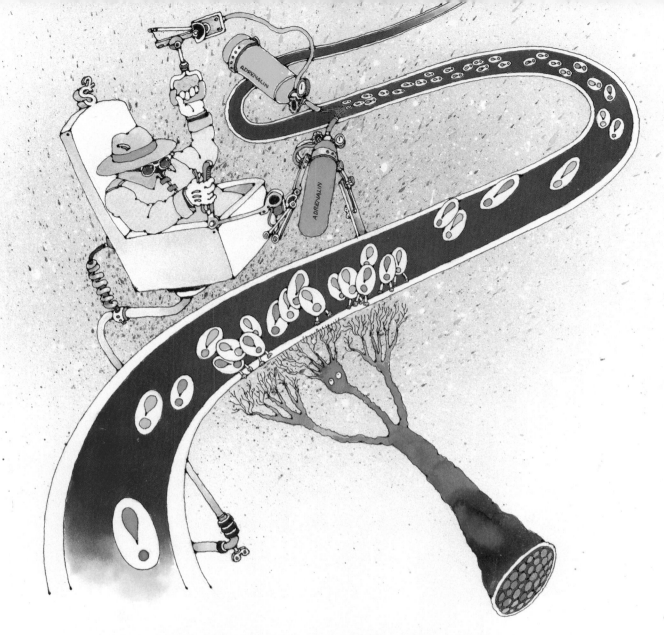

"Ah…lungs breathing harder…more oxygen for the blood-stream. Let's see…the liver is putting extra sugar into the blood.

Good…extra energy going where it's needed. Stomach…we need your blood elsewhere." The stomach turns from red to pink as the blood is suddenly drained away, moving toward the muscles in the arms and legs.

"Now the heart," says the Inspector. "Excellent! Beating much harder and faster. That'll get all the extra fuel and energy to the muscles for quick action."

Suddenly the entire Land of U lurches backward so fast that the Inspector falls off his stool. Leg muscles have suddenly changed direction.

The Inspector checks out the situation in the Great Beyond. The car and the land of U have both screeched to a halt. The Land of U has stepped backward. The ball is on the other side of the street. Clearly, the emergency is over and no damage has been done.

But it could have been worse. A lot worse. The Inspector smiles and reaches for the Axon Messenger Service.

"Get me the Autonomic Nervous System, Parasympathetic Division. Hello, Vagus Nerve? Danger is over. You can resume normal operations. Tell your other half to take a rest."

"We're happy to do so," answers Vagus. "I think the Sympathetic Division performed so well that we're going to sing it a lullabye."

The Inspector listens as the Parasympathetic Division croons to its partner as they take control over different parts of the nation's functioning and return things to normal.

> Danger's past, go back to resting,
> Our Sympathetic friend.
> When the threat came, you did the best thing
> Right to the end.
> You made the heart pound faster,
> The lungs breathe deeper,
> The blood gets richer,
> The muscles stronger.
> Now it's our turn, back to normal
> Lucky us, there're no wounds to mend.

Inspector Bodyguard smiles with satisfaction at the Parasympathetic lullabye. Things are calm enough for the Inspector to grab some shut-eye himself. He settles back in his chair, closes his eyes and naps. His dreams are peaceful.

HOW YOUR BODY REACTS TO SUDDEN DANGER

When danger strikes, survival often depends on moving quickly and being able to keep functioning even if you are injured. At a dangerous moment, there is often no time to think. So the body has a built-in emergency system that takes over and automatically prepares you for the worst. Here's how it works.

The first part of your reaction is the startle reflex. Like all reflexes, the startle reflex is a reaction to some outside event (such as a car horn) that your nervous system responds to without using your brain. A reflex always has the same pattern and happens in less than half a second. The part of the nervous system that is used for the startle reflex is the *autonomic nervous system*.

The autonomic nervous system controls the functioning of the inner organs of the body, including the heart, lungs, and digestive system. There are two divisions to the autonomic nervous system, which have opposite effects on various organs. Both divisions are connected to a part of your brain called the *hypothalamus*. The hypothalamus is involved in your emotions as well as the autonomic nervous system. The *parasympathetic* division is responsible for making saliva and keeping digestion going. It also slows down rapid heart and breathing rates. The *sympathetic* division is active during danger or anger. Here is the chain of events that went on in the last Inspector Bodyguard story.

The car horn is detected by the ear and translated into a nerve impulse that travels along incoming sympathetic nerves at about one hundred miles per hour. The incoming nerves meet outgoing sympathetic nerves at *ganglia* located along the outside of the spinal cord. The outgoing nerves produce the movements connected with the startle reflex that everybody—but everybody from babies to old people—does exactly the same way. Your eyes close, your head tips forward, your shoulders tighten and hunch over, you take a giant breath and bend forward in a bow as your knees start to crouch. This position protects your eyes and your vital organs while your legs get in position to spring away. Inside, outgoing sympathetic nerves stimulate the *adrenal medulla* glands, located in your back on top of your kidneys.

By this time, you've opened your eyes and seen the danger. The adrenal medulla pours adrenalin into your bloodstream. As adrenaline is pumped around the body it comes in contact with the ends of the sympathetic nervous system

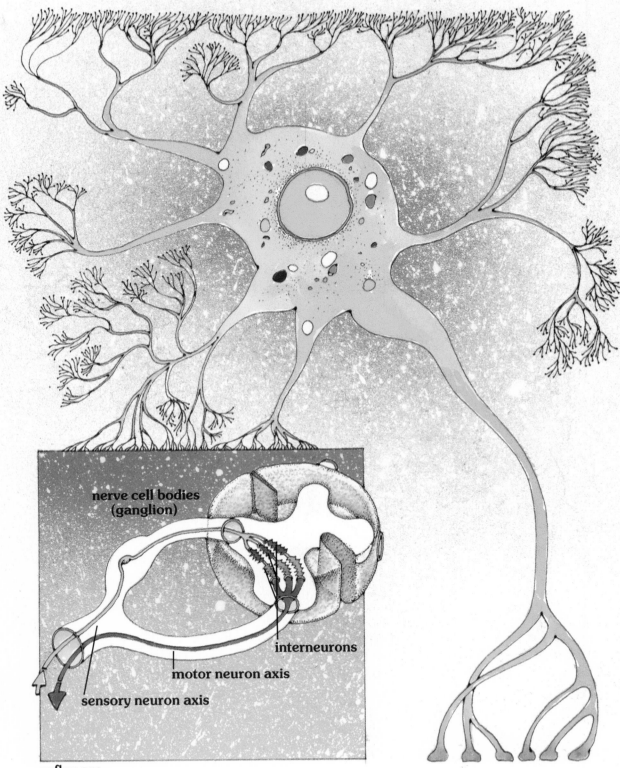

nerve cell bodies
(ganglion)

interneurons

motor neuron axis

sensory neuron axis

reflex arc

in various organs. The effect of adrenalin on sympathetic nerves is powerful and instantaneous, like an electric shock. The activated nerves make the organs respond immediately in ways that help you survive the danger.

Your skin pales and you get "white with fright" as the blood vessels near the surface constrict. This diverts the blood supply to the inner organs where it's needed and lessens the chance of heavy bleeding if your skin is cut. Digestion stops as blood is diverted from the stomach to the heart, liver and lungs. Saliva secretion stops, leaving your mouth feeling dry. The purpose of all these changes is to prepare you to move quickly, to "take flight" and get out of the way if that is the proper response. If the danger is an attack by an animal you are also prepared to fight. You are frozen motionless as your brain starts to understand what's happening and decides whether flight or fight is the proper response.

The powerful and unpleasant feelings generated by your built-in "flight or fight" reaction helps you remember the painful lesson of a near miss. If you have had this kind of experience, you can become afraid just by running into the street without looking. There doesn't have to be a car present to remind you that you might be in danger.

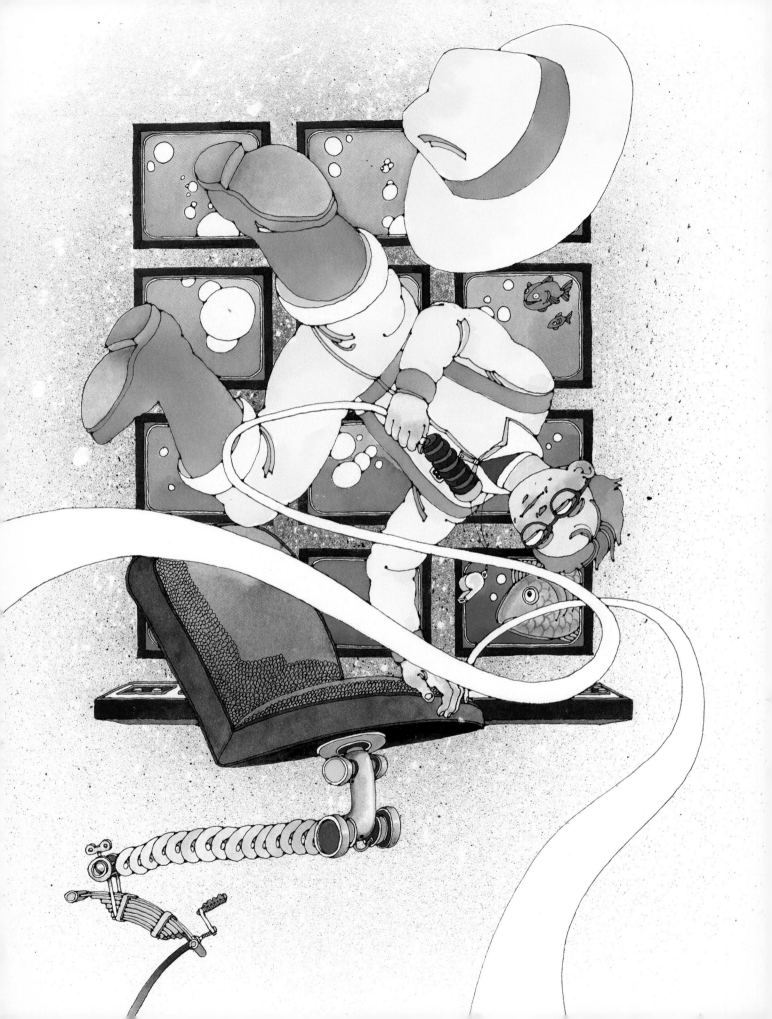

5:

FIGHTING THE BIG CHILL

Inspector Bodyguard moves quickly into his chair in Cortex Central and straps on his seatbelt. He feels himself moving up and then, suddenly, he is upside down. A moment later, and the entire Land of U shakes briefly. Then, all is calm. The Inspector unbelts himself, enjoying an almost weightless feeling. The Land of U has just dived into a swimming pool and is now having fun in the water.

The Inspector knows from experience that the Land of U is not likely to be on dry land again for a long time. Normally, the Land of U has red lips and blue eyes. But after an hour or so in the pool, he will have blue lips and red eyes. A cool pool is not the normal environment for the Land of U. Too much time in the water has certain dangers. Inspector Bodyguard knows he must be on his toes.

First things, first. The Inspector decides to stop in at Hypothala-

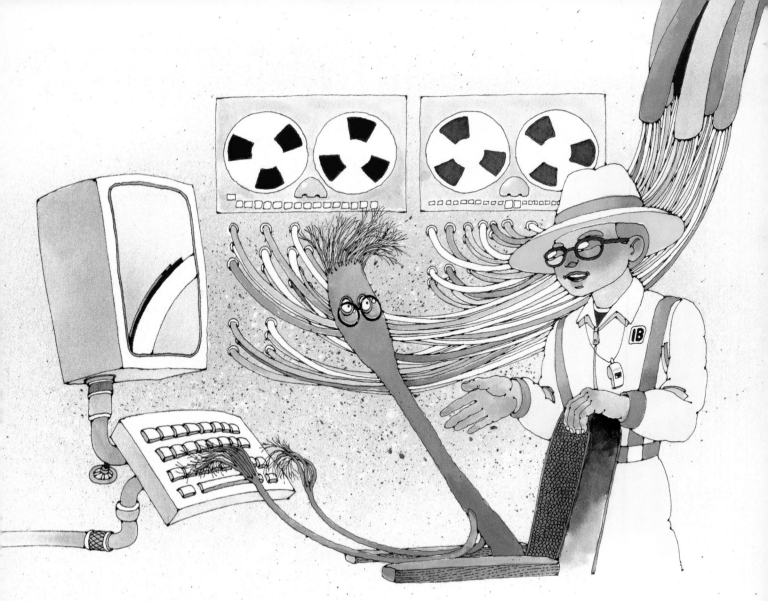

mus Computer Base. It is the big switchboard for incoming messages from the Great Beyond to the Autonomic Nervous System.

"How's the automatic thermostat, Chief?" Inspector Bodyguard asks the HCB manager, Chief Underbrain, who is peering at the controls.

"Oh, hi, Inspector. It looks as if we're going to be losing a lot of heat. The water temperature is about 75 degrees and the Land of U is normally 98.6 degrees. Yep! We can count on that heat loss," answers the Chief.

"It looks as if our problem, as per usual, will be Brain Command Post with a mind of his own. Somehow we have to get it through Brain's thick skull that a heat loss can create a serious situation for the entire Land of U." The Inspector shakes his head in disgust.

When it comes to overdoing things while having fun, Brain never seems to learn his lesson.

"Well, I'll start by sending a message through the Sympathetic branch to close down the small blood vessels near Skin Frontier."

"Good thinking, Chief. I'll go check the response at Lipskin Passage. The results of the cutback on blood should be quite clear there. If nothing else, causing blue lips will alert someone in The Great Beyond that the Land of U is losing heat."

"It's true that this action doesn't do very much by itself. But it keeps the blood deeper in the Land of U, away from the surface where heat is lost most quickly. At best, it lets us stay in the cold longer. It doesn't generate any new heat, just slows down the rate at which we lose it," says Chief Underbrain. "And oh, Inspector, before I forget. You'd better check the morale of all the Hairy Pilis. They've been complaining lately. They think their job is useless. But they've still got to do it. They'll be getting my order to go to work next."

"Okay, Chief. I'll do that. Keep those nerves firing." The Inspector steps into his Blood Buggy for a trip to Lipskin Passage.

On this trip the Inspector is too preoccupied to notice the smoothly flowing traffic of Red Cell Truckers and the occasional patrolling Germbuster that travel with him along Jugular Turnpike. The Blood Buggy passes flattened valves that prevent the flow from backing up and changing direction in case the land of U is upside down. At about the level of Tongue Receiving Station, the Inspector turns off Jugular Turnpike into a small capillary that will deliver him to the ridge of Upper Lip.

Inspector Bodyguard hops off and wanders among the capillaries at Lipskin Passage.

"We got the message, Inspector," calls Cappy Capillary. "We've pulled in our walls. But Lipskin cells are using up all the oxygen in the Red Cell Truckers. Our blood is turning blue. And so is Lipskin."

"That's the idea, Cappy. You know blood always turns blue when it doesn't have its full share of oxygen. So Lipskin Passage is blue.

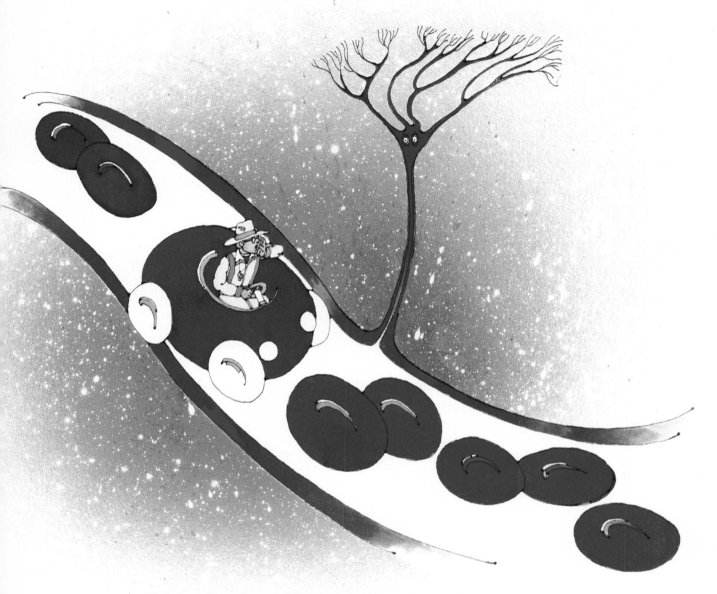

The condition is temporary. The color will return to red when we get out of this pool and warm up. You can open up then, Cappy. Bring in lots of oxygen-heavy, warm, fresh Truckers. But until you get the sign, keep cool and closed." The first stage of the Heat Conservation Operation is in effect. The Inspector gets back into the Blood Buggy and decides to meet with the cranky Hairy Pilis in the Skin Frontier of the Great Chest Plain.

The Hairy Pilis are small muscles that have the job of making hair stand on end. When the Land of U is losing heat, they have to pull, pull hard, and keep pulling. By this time in a big chill, they are in their clenched position. The Inspector can hear the chorus of their complaint as he draws near.

During cold weather
in each lion and bear
We make their fur warmer
as we hoist up each hair.

When fur stands at attention
it traps extra air
Which acts as a blanket
as we hoist up each hair.

But there's no fur on people.

Their skin is quite bare.
We pull our weight anyhow
and hoist up each hair.

We hoist when it's chilly
and when there's a scare.
We make goose bumps, not blankets
as we hoist up each hair.

Goose bumps can't help U.
We don't think that's fair.
Without fur, it's still work
to hoist up each hair.

But we're tied to tradition.
Quit? We don't dare.
Our job seems quite useless,
Still, we hoist up each hair.

Inspector Bodyguard shakes his head in amusement. What can he do about their feeling of uselessness? Most workers want to know their job is meaningful. He sighs to himself, then pulls out his whistle and blows for attention.

"Hairy Pilis, my friends, don't ruffle your feathers. So what if human hair isn't woolly and thick! When you pull together you make skin know that it's cold. That's an important warning for Brain Command Post. BCP can get the Land of U to cover up, go where it's warmer. Don't feel unneeded. Suppose you didn't do your job. How would the Land of U know it was losing heat? He would have to wait for heat generating shakes. Your action can

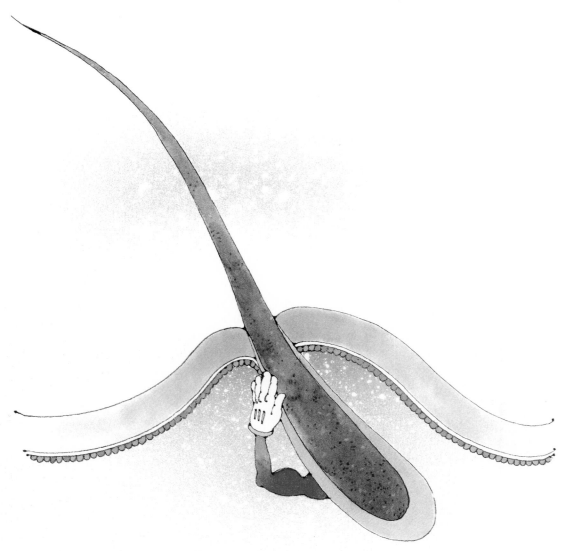

cut heat loss short. So I say to each of you, 'Keep it up, whether it's your good work or your spirits!' "

"That's just what we do, Inspector. Keep it up." A Hairy Pili eyes his hair, which he is holding in a vertical position. The Skin Frontier around the hair is puckered into a mound. At least this Hairy Pili is making a respectable goose bump.

The Inspector waves goodbye and gets back into the Blood Buggy. It's clear that the messages from the goose bumps and blue lips are not getting through to Brain Command Post. The Land of U is still happily swimming in the pool. The heat loss is increasing every moment. It's time for the next step, the drastic one. The Land of U will have to start making heat before it gets much colder. Inspector Bodyguard turns the Blood Buggy and heads for Tongue Receiving Station. That's a good place to check on the Heat Generating Process.

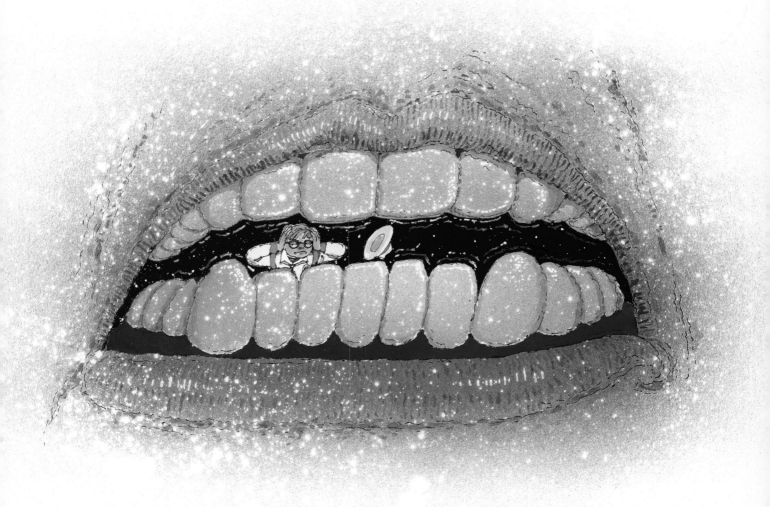

Inspector Bodyguard puts in a call to Chief Underbrain. "Is body temperature holding, Chief? Or are we still losing heat?"

"We're down a degree, Inspector. It's time to start phase three of our Heat Conservation Operation. Muscles have got to start moving rapidly. Moving muscles generate heat. I hope you're standing clear in Mouth Terminal, Inspector." Chief Underbrain throws the switch to start involuntary muscle spasms, also called shivering.

Inspector Bodyguard puts his hands over his ears as the jaw muscles start working and the back molars crash together. Chattering teeth give the Inspector a loud measure of how much shivering is taking place.

"That ought to get the Land of U out of the water," mutters the Inspector. The noise in Mouth Terminal is deafening. The Land of U burns fuel to move its muscles. Some of the energy used to move muscles is also given off as heat. But if the Land of U doesn't get somewhere warm soon, shivering alone cannot restore body temperature to normal. At best, it can only slow down the cooling process. And the Inspector knows that severe, deep cooling can ultimately cause unconsciousness.

Suddenly, the Inspector feels himself get heavy again. He breathes a sigh of relief, "Nerves preserve us...the Land of U is acting sensibly. We're out of the water. Normal temperature can be restored...until the next time the Land of U decides to go swimming."

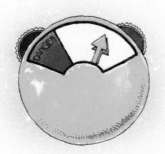

HOW YOUR BODY FIGHTS A CHILL

Most of the animals on earth, the insects, fish, snakes, and frogs, have body temperatures that are the same as the air or water surrounding them. If it's cold out, they're cold. If it's warm, they're warm. The activities of such "cold-blooded" creatures depend on the weather. When it is cold, they live and move more slowly than when it is warm.

On the other hand, birds and mammals can maintain the same body temperature independent of how warm or cold it is outside, up to a point. Birds keep heat from escaping by a covering of feathers. Mammals keep from losing heat with a blanket of fur or a layer of fat under the skin. For this reason, mammals and birds live in all parts of the world, not just places that are comfortably warm. And their activity does not depend so much on the outside temperature.

Your normal body temperature is about 98.6 degrees Fahrenheit. It is kept at this temperature by the *hypothalamus*, a small body about the size of a finger located under your brain behind your nose in the center of your head. The hypothalamus acts like a switchboard connecting the *sympathetic* and *parasympathetic nervous systems*. When you are cold, the hypothalamus turns on the sympathetic nervous system to help you lose heat more slowly.

The first step is to cause all the surface blood vessels to contract. This keeps the blood, which is always moving around the body, away from the surface, where it cools off most quickly. Most of the blood is now in the body's core, where heat is lost more slowly. The blood that is left behind near the skin quickly loses its oxygen to the nearby cells. Blood that has lost oxygen is bluish in color. This blue blood is especially noticeable where the skin is thin. That's why your lips turn blue with cold.

Next, the small muscles that attach to each body hair contract. These muscles, called *arrector pilis*, make goose bumps when they raise each hair. In furry animals, they make fur stand on end, trapping extra air, insulation which preserves body heat. In human beings, goose bumps don't really do this very well. Our body hair is too thin. It may be left behind from some ancestor who had much more body hair. Clothing does the job of fur.

When muscles work, they use energy and give off more heat than when they are resting. Long, drawn out physical activity can raise body temperature.

INSPECTOR BODYGUARD

When you lose a lot of heat to colder surroundings, your hypothalamus makes your muscles move without your control. You shiver. Your teeth chatter. This extra motion can make you warmer. But if your surroundings are really cold, shivering only slows down how fast you get chilled. It can't really raise your body temperature until you get to a warmer place.

As your body loses heat, your arms and legs get cold first. If the skin of your hands drops to 60 degrees, they will feel numb. When they warm up, you may feel intense pain. As your body temperature gets lower, you shiver. But shiver-

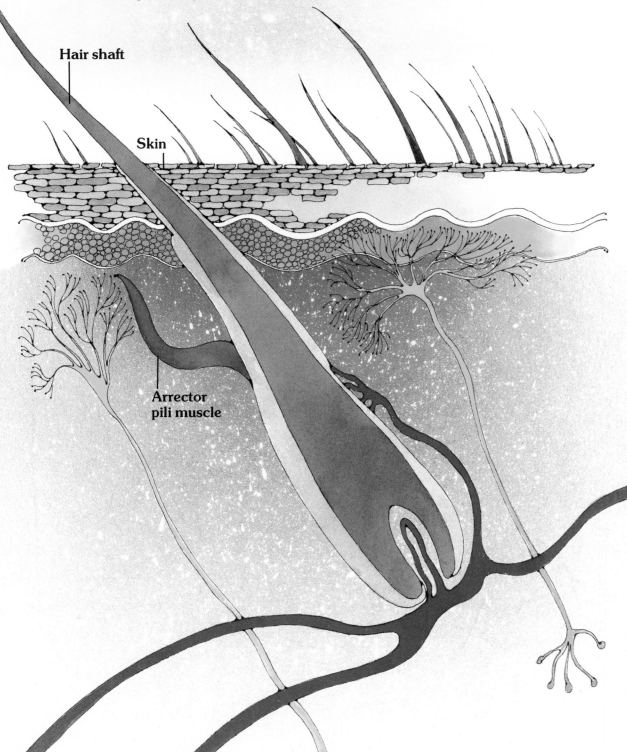

Hair shaft

Skin

Arrector pili muscle

ing stops if your core temperature cools to 90 degrees. At this temperature your muscles get stiff and you are likely to pass out. You start breathing more slowly and your heart no longer has a steady beat. The heart stops beating at about 75 degrees.

Can you survive deep cooling? Freezing of parts of the body causes frostbite. The blood supply to frostbitten tissues is cut off and there is not enough oxygen getting to the cells to keep them alive. If frostbite is very severe, the tissue will die. Long exposure to the outdoors in freezing weather can produce conditions of very low core body temperatures. Professional medical treatment is important for a person who has suffered such exposure. There have been some amazing stories of people who have survived deep cooling. But it's not an experience anyone would want to risk having.

6:

RED RIVER FLOOD AT SKIN FRONTIER

As Keeper of the Health, it is Inspector Bodyguard's job to patrol the Land of U at least once a day. The Inspector likes to visit different cell citizens and make sure everyone feels well. On this particular day the Inspector can hear the fine humming of alpha waves from Brain Command Post. The Inspector knows that alpha waves mean that BCP is at peace, working at its highest level. The Land of U is functioning well in the Great Beyond. What can be going on? While on patrol, the Inspector stops by Pupil Park for a look. From Pupil Park he can see the part of the Land of U that connects with the Great Beyond.

"Happy hormones! The Land of U is being creative today down at Hands' End. What are we making? Is it a bird? Is it a plane? It could be either. It's made from wood, and Hands' End is carving it. I can't wait to see what it will be."

The Inspector gazes happily at the working hands. The penknife

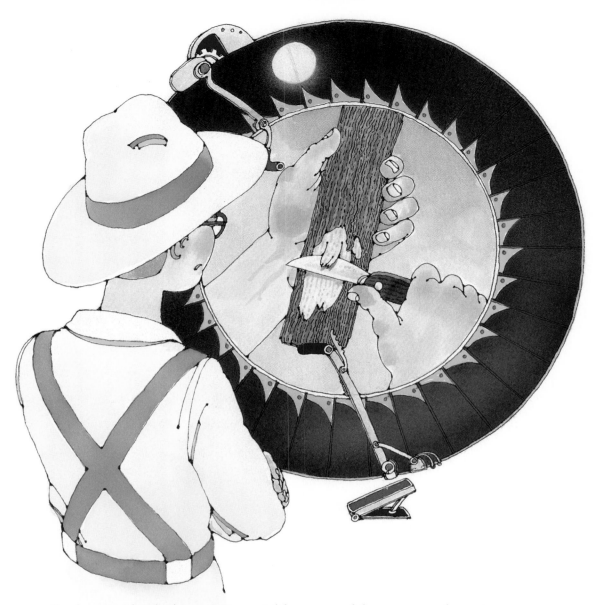

flashes in the light as it is quickly moved from one place to another. Chips are flying. The Inspector feels the alpha waves coming from Brain Command Post make beautiful music. It's clear that the Land of U is completely involved in his activity.

Then, right before the Inspector's horrified eyes, the knife slips and cuts Left Index Finger. Instantly there is a crimson flood all over the carving as Red River is released through the cut skin. The Inspector can hear the cries of the injured cells of Skin Frontier.

Hands' End drops the knife and the carving. A howl comes from the back of Mouth Receiving Station. The alpha waves from Brain Command Post have been replaced by beta waves. Brain is clearly feeling pain.

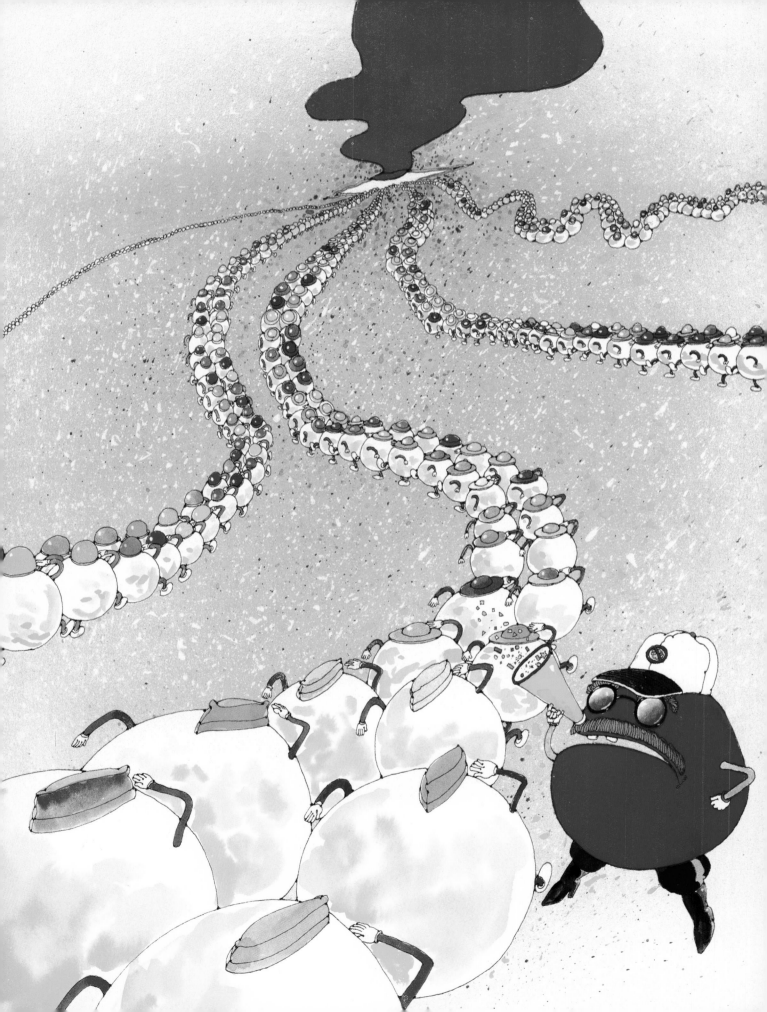

"Axon Messenger Service, get me Captain Blast," phones the Inspector. "There is no time to waste. The leak is not huge, but it must be stopped." The Inspector does not like to lose a drop of the Land of U's precious Red River.

"Right here, Inspector," comes the calm, controlled voice of Captain Blast, the top officer of all the blood cell citizens. "I'm at the flood, ready to call the shots until you get here. You hopping the Blood Buggy?"

"I'm on my way. Better give the green light to the platelets to call them to duty. Command them to march forward,"

"Will do, Inspector." Captain Blast turns toward the rushing river. He shouts to the millions of platelets moving before him, "Okay boys...Get in there and plug!"

The platelets begin chanting their march to battle.

> Plug! Plug! Plug! Plug!
> Plug! Plug! Plug! Plug!
> Onward platelets! Onward platelets!
> Marching to the flood.
>
> Caused by a slip of a knife
> A definite threat to life.
> We stick together at the injury site
> Making a dam, we start to fight.
>
> For we're the clotting army of the blood.
> Plug! Plug! Plug!
> Plug! Plug! Plug! Plug!
>
> Onward platelets! Onward platelets!
> We're pros in chemical war.
>
> Our powerful juices do a lot
> In the formation of a clot.
> They shrink blood vessels very small
> And help make threads to build a wall.
>
> We fight to stop blood flowing at the sore.
> Plug! Plug! Plug!
> Plug! Plug! Plug! Plug!

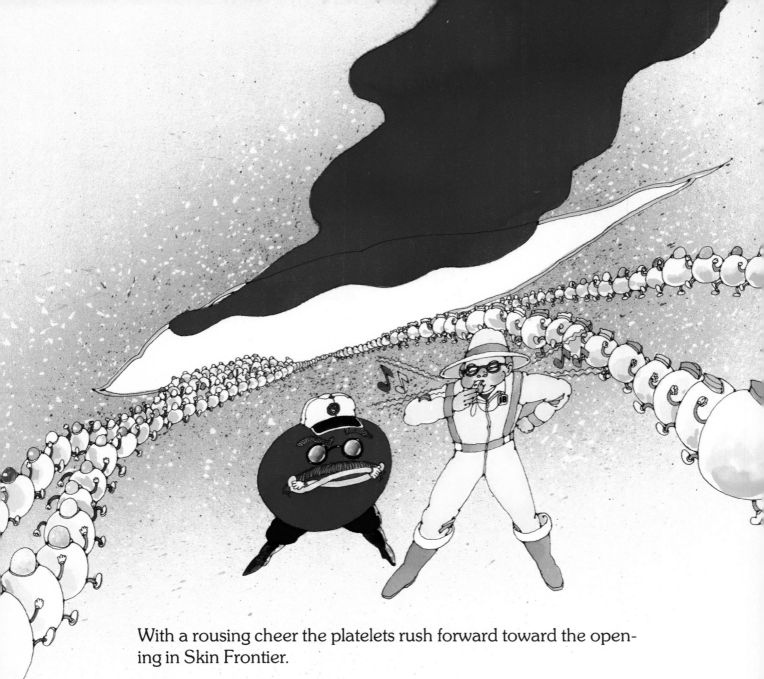

With a rousing cheer the platelets rush forward toward the opening in Skin Frontier.

The Inspector arrives just as the platelets start piling up along the injured cells. They are forming a temporary dam to slow the flow. But more help is needed. Inspector Bodyguard blows his whistle for attention.

"Wounded citizens of Fingerprint Ridge, we must put Plasma Defense Plan into action to stop the loss of any more of the Red River. If you are dying, remember how you were trained. You must release your thrombobombs as a last gesture. Your lives are over. Do this for those who must live on."

"Good speech, Inspector," says Captain Blast. "This is a time when those who are doomed must act to protect the living. Very unselfish of them."

They watch as countless thrombobombs are released into the blood plasma, the clear liquid that is the main part of the Red River.

"Things should now be pretty automatic," comments Inspector Bodyguard.

"Yep!" says the Captain. "Those thrombobombs are the trigger that sets off a pretty spectacular chain of events. The platelets have also added their part to the mix. I love watching what happens. It's like fireworks on the Fourth of July."

Indeed, a spectacular sight meets their eyes. The thrombobombs from the dying cells and juices released by the platelets mix to form a powerful chemical. This chemical meets up with invisible coiled balls that have been floating all along in the clear blood plasma. Zap! and each coiled ball springs open, forming a long thread. Suddenly there are threads everywhere, going in every direction. A tangled network acts as a fishnet, catching blood cells as they float by.

"Help! Help! I'm trapped!" yells a Red Cell Trucker.

"My job carrying oxygen is over, alas!" cries another.

"We'll add color to the clot," says a third, resigned to his fate.

"Sacrifices can't be avoided," says the Inspector to them in a soothing voice. "You'll be a part of the scab that will protect the wound as it heals. You'll help keep out germs. You'll be important even after you're dead."

As the network of threads becomes complete, the spaces are filled with millions of trapped red and white blood cells. Suddenly the net tightens, squeezing out a clear fluid.

"The scab is now complete, Inspector," says Captain Blast. "Serum has just been released. Now the scab will harden and act as a protective skin."

"Yes. The scab will get tough, just like dead skin cells. Under-

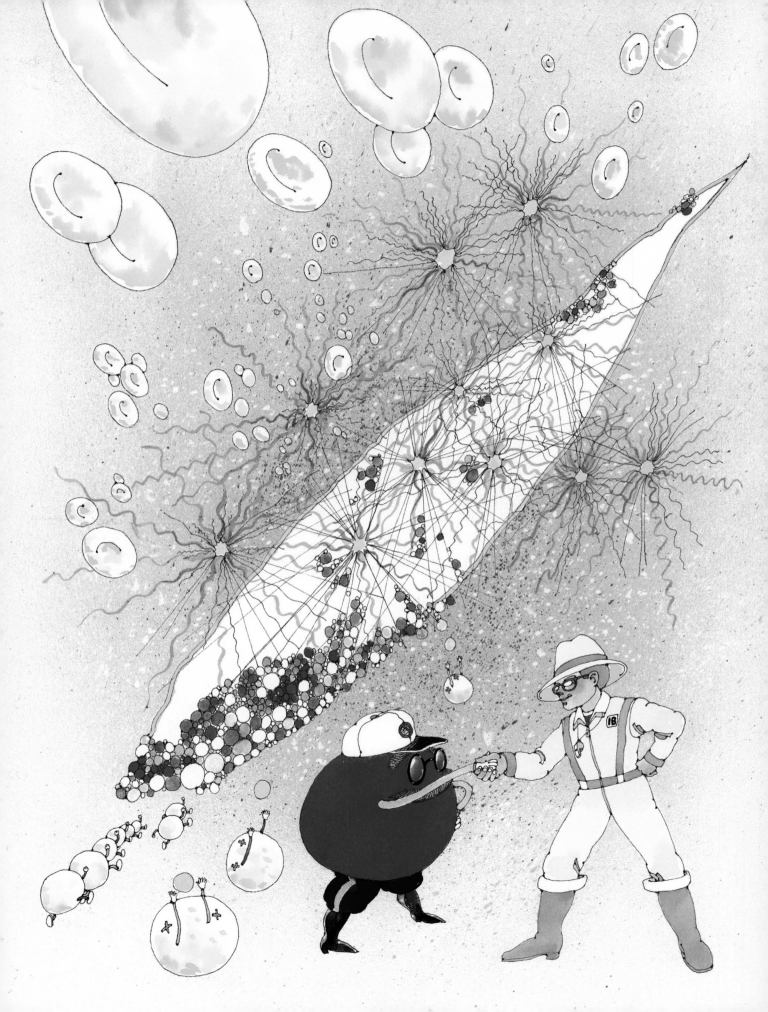

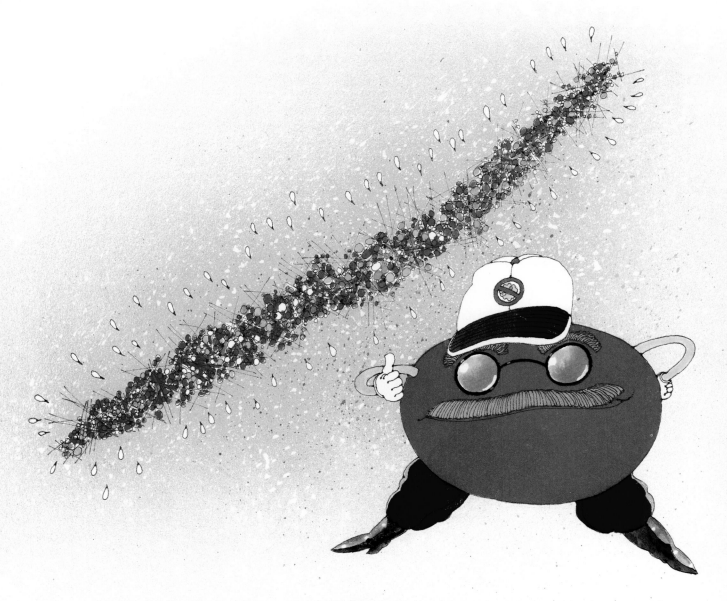

neath, the cells of Skin Frontier will have a chance to grow and repair the damage. The flood of the Red River is now dammed up.
When the repair is complete, the scab will come off. It will have
done its job to perfection. I hate to think what would happen to
the Land of U if blood didn't clot so quickly."

"It's quite simple, Inspector. We would never survive. Even a
small cut could do us in."

"Well, the perfection of all the systems in the Land of U certainly
make our jobs easy, Captain."

The Inspector and Captain shake hands as they congratulate
each other on another successfully completed mission in the
Land of U.

HOW
YOUR BLOOD CLOTS TO STOP BLEEDING

Your body has between four and five quarts of blood when you are full grown. Depending on your age, you can lose about one quart without serious consequences. But if you lose more than a quart of blood your body suffers severely. Blood has the all-important job of delivering oxygen to all parts of the body. When you lose a lot of blood, the tissues of the body don't get enough oxygen. You go into a condition called *shock*.

When you are in shock, your blood vessels can't be properly filled. Your blood pressure drops and your heart speeds up, trying to keep the blood moving where it's needed. You feel weak and cold and break out in a cold sweat. You feel thirsty and gasp for breath. If you don't get a blood transfusion, you may become unconscious.

You don't lose a lot of blood from ordinary cuts and bruises because your blood has a built-in means of plugging leaks. There is a protein called *fibrinogen* that is dissolved in the blood plasma, the clear, watery fluid of the blood. (Blood gets its red color from the billions of red blood cells that actually do the job of carrying oxygen. They are the "red cell truckers" in the stories.) Fibrinogen becomes a threadlike protein, called *fibrin*, that doesn't dissolve. Fibrin threads are the network that forms a blood clot and eventually a scab.

Obviously, you can't have blood clots forming inside blood vessels. There are certain diseases where blood clots do form in arteries and veins and cause all kinds of problems. Clots block the flow of blood. Such a blockage in a blood vessel that nourishes the heart causes a heart attack. A blockage that prevents blood from reaching the brain causes a stroke. The problem the body solves is how to have dissolved fibrinogen *everywhere* in the blood ready to become fibrin threads, but *only* when the situation calls for it. The solution is that fibrinogen can't become fibrin without a trigger. So under normal conditions the blood is fluid, without clots.

Injury and bleeding are the proper times for blood to clot. The trigger that reacts with fibrinogen to form fibrin is a substance called *thrombin*. To further protect the body against accidental clots, the thrombin has to be put together from a number of pieces present in the platelets and in the plasma. A chain of events does this where there's a cut. Here's what happens.

In every drop of blood there are at least fifteen million platelets, truly the clotting army of the blood. First, platelets start sticking to the walls of the injured blood vessels and to each other, forming a temporary plug that slows the loss of blood.

Both the injured cells and the platelets give off a chemical that causes the wounded blood vessels to contract. This slows the blood flow from the wound. The platelets also give off another chemical that combines with blood proteins to form thrombin. All in all, there are more than a dozen different factors that play a part in forming thrombin. When a thrombin molecule meets a fibrinogen molecule, a string of fibrin is the instant reaction. It all happens quite quickly. In the case of a small cut, the fibrin appears about two minutes after the injury.

bleeding   **clot forming**

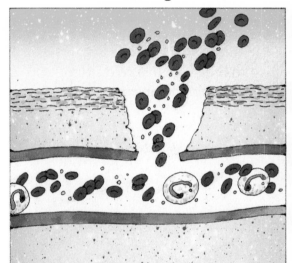 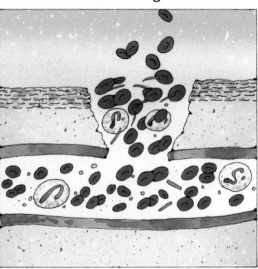

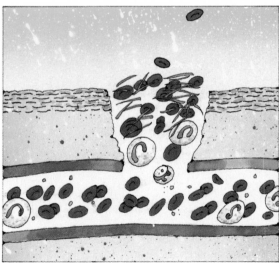 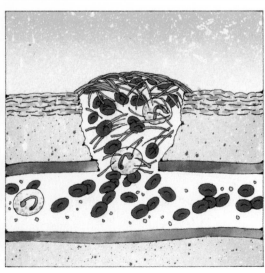

fibrin released   **fibrin forms scab**

At first, the fibrin strands are quite stretched out. They form a network that traps millions of red blood cells, giving the clot its typical red color. Then they shrink, squeezing out a clear yellowish liquid. This is blood *serum*. Serum is blood plasma that has all of the clotting material removed. When a blood clot is on the skin, exposed to the air, it gradually toughens and gets harder in much the same way skin gets tough. A hardened blood clot on the skin becomes a *scab*. The scab remains over the wound while the skin repairs itself. New cells replace those destroyed by the injury. White blood cells clean up debris left behind by bacteria. When the damage has been repaired, the scab falls off, having done its job.

Uncontrolled bleeding is called a *hemorrhage*. Severe bleeding from an arm or leg can be controlled by applying pressure on the side of the wound closer to the heart. This squeezes the blood vessels closed and shuts down the flow. Some dangerous hemorrhages occur inside the body and can't be seen. Such internal bleeding is usually caused by a serious injury. Surgeons often enter the body to close the wound causing the bleeding. Blood transfusions are given when a lot of blood has been lost.

There are people known as "bleeders," or *hemophiliacs*, whose blood clots very slowly or not at all. Hemophilia is inherited mostly by sons from their mothers. Hemophiliacs must live very carefully, trying to avoid minor injuries because even a small cut can be fatal. Hemophiliacs bleed because a protein important for blood clotting is missing from their blood. Today, hemophiliacs can inject this protein into their blood and live nearly normal lives.

7:

A DANGEROUS, HOT, DRY SPELL

Inspector Bodyguard wakes up with the land of U. Things have been going extremely well lately. The Land of U is on summer vacation and there have been enjoyable activities everyday.

"I wonder what the plan is for today," muses the Inspector. "Shall I tune in Brain and see what's on Brain's mind? Maybe I'll just wait and see what comes." The Inspector rolls over and closes his eyes. He feels as if he's on vacation, also. In the distance, filtering through from the Great Beyond, he hears the weather forecast.

"Today's going to be a scorcher. Expect sunny skies, slightly overcast with temperatures...are you ready for this?...near the 100 degree mark! Humidity will also be up. Today is one of those days to lie low. No wonder they call it a 'Dog Day' of summer."

"Mmmmmm, I'd better check in with Chief Underbrain at Hypothalamus Computer Base...Adjustments will have to be made today..."

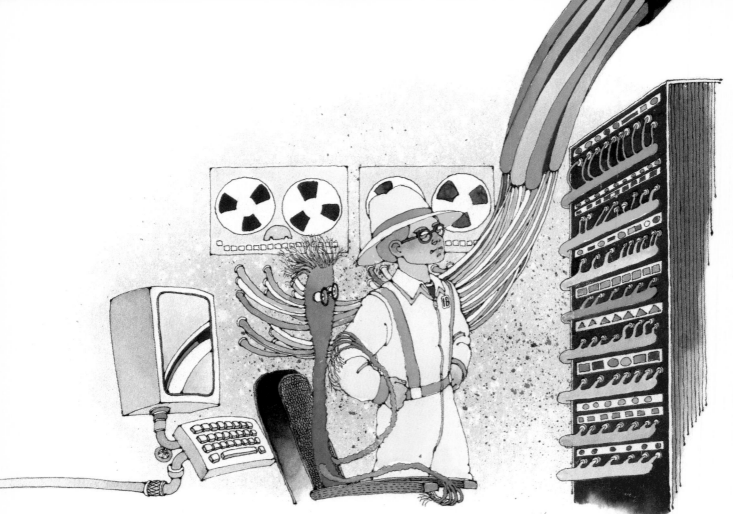

The Inspector feels the activity starting as the Land of U bounces out of bed and gets ready for the day. The heat certainly isn't slowing him down yet.

An hour later the Inspector is in the Hypothalamus Computer Base. Chief Underbrain is involved in watching the incoming messages from Skin Frontier. The Inspector silently watches with him for a few minutes.

"The switchboard is busy this morning, Chief. We're already getting information from all parts of the Land of U."

"There will be a lot of action here today, Inspector. We're just about to do something about the rising temperatures on Skin Frontier. That's the message I'm getting loud and clear from the entire nation."

"When are you alerting the Sympathetic Division?" asks the Inspector.

"Right now. Want to throw the switch?"

Inspector Bodyguard nods and clicks on the switch that sends the response along the wires of the Sympathetic Division to the entire Skin Frontier.

"That should cool things off," says Chief Underbrain with satisfaction.

"Yes…well…you carry on here, Chief. I think I'll pay a visit to Skin Frontier. The sweat glands on Forehead Plain are usually among the first to react. I'll just make sure they got the message and are stepping up sweat production. See you later."

But the Chief is totally involved with his work. He has returned to his monitors and pays no attention to the departing Inspector, who is stepping into his Blood Buggy for a trip to Forehead Plain.

As the Inspector nears his destination, he notices that the surroundings have become redder than usual.

"Good!" he thinks to himself. "All the capillaries are open. More blood is being shipped to the surface for cooling before returning to the nation's heartland."

Like many of the workers in the Land of U, the sweat glands sing a worksong as they do their job. Inspector Bodyguard smiles to himself as he feels their enthusiasm for their job.

> Dripity high! Dripity low!
> When hot skin has a rosy glow
> We make clothes stick from head to toe
> To cool U off when breezes blow.
> Dripity high! Dripity low!
>
> Dripity less! Dripity more!
> When temperatures rise in the body's core,
> We squirt our juice through every pore.
> We're two million strong. That's sweat galore!
> Dripity less! Dripity more!
>
> Dripity early! Dripity late!
> Our fluids make U regulate
> The body's salt and water state.
> For it's waste we help eliminate.
> Dripity early! Dripity late!

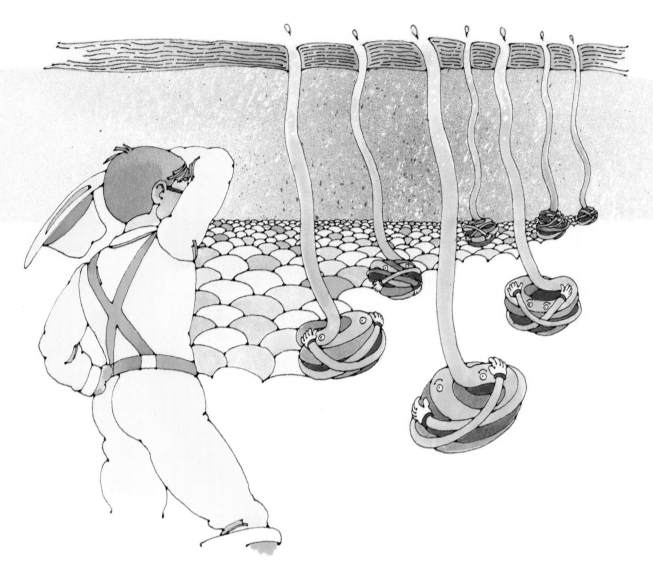

The Inspector watches in fascination as a tiny muscle squeezes the coiled tube at the bottom of a sweat gland. A bead of sweat quickly travels up the tube through a pore on the surface of Forehead Plain, where it shoots out like a miniature geyser. The bead of sweat glistens there for a few minutes before it evaporates. Inspector Bodyguard knows that some of the heat in the skin is used up to evaporate the sweat. That's how sweat does its job of cooling off the body. The sweat production satisfies him that the right messages have been received from Chief Underbrain.

Suddenly, the entire Land of U becomes quite active. The motion makes it hard for the Inspector to keep his balance. The sweat glands become busier than ever.

"Salty sweat glands! What's going on? I'd better take a look from

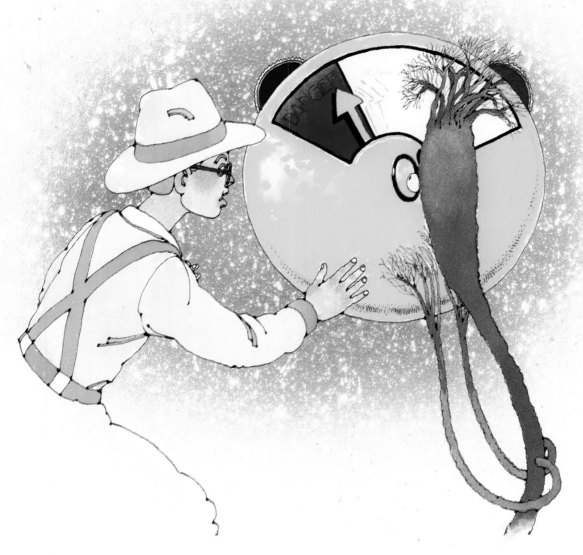

Pupil Park. Good thing it's not far from here." The Inspector hops back into his Blood Buggy.

The minute he peers out into the Great Beyond from Pupil Park, it is very clear what's happening. "Great suffering synapses! The Land of U is involved in a very heated tennis match. And in this weather! Sometimes I think Brain doesn't care about the well-being of the rest of the Land of U. Doesn't it know that activity creates even more heat? Dumb Brain!"

The Inspector shakes his head worriedly. "This doesn't look good for our nation's water supply," he mutters to himself. "The sweat glands are going to need more than their share. I'd better get back to Computer Base. We need this kind of activity today like the ocean needs salt."

With a determined look on his face, the Inspector makes his journey back to Hypothalamus Computer Base. It's going to be a long day. He can feel it in his bones. It's time for him to take charge as Keeper of the Health of the land of U.

"Put the Water Conservation Program into effect, Chief. The sweat glands are going to drain the Red River as much as they can."

"Right! Inspector," Chief Underbrain says, getting ready to throw switches.

"Cut down water going into the liquid waste at the Kidney Filtering Plant."

"You got it, Inspector!"

"Make less water available for saliva. That ought to create a parched condition at Mouth Terminal. Make the Land of U thirsty enough to import water from the Great Beyond."

Chief Underbrain throws another switch. "Done, Inspector...Er ...I hate to mention this, but what if we don't get water pretty soon?"

"We'd better. The Land of U will feel very uncomfortable without it. Hey! Maybe we're getting some now."

Inspector Bodyguard and Chief Underbrain hold their breath, listening for signs from the Great Beyond. But they don't hear the familiar slurping that indicates an intake of water.

Inspector Bodyguard and Chief Underbrain look at each other and groan. The Water Conservation Program will be strained to the utmost.

"Let's not forget," says the Inspector, "that we're also losing salt along with water. We could be in for an extreme case of dehydration or heat stroke. Chief, I may have to take drastic action."

The Keeper of the Health settles into a corner of the Computer Base to wait for the Land of U to do what is necessary. The hours tick by. The Land of U shows no sign of stopping his activity, getting out of the sun, or getting a drink. Finally the Inspector stands

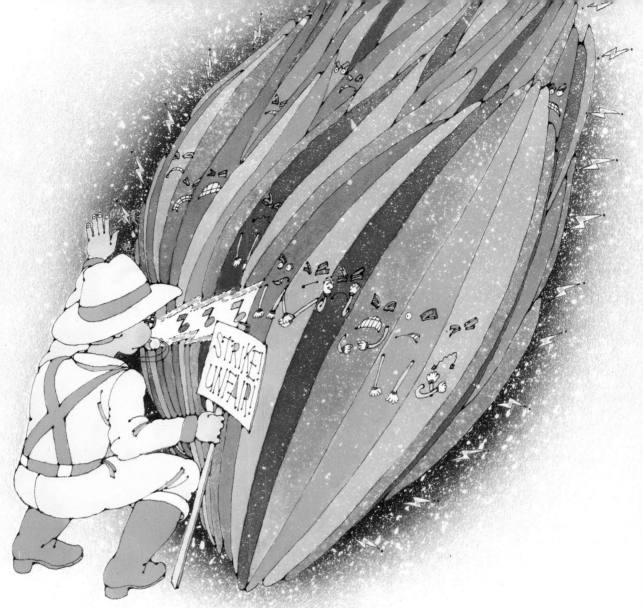

up and says, "I've had enough of this. I'll make him stop."
Purposefully, the Inspector gets in the Blood Buggy and directs it
towards Great Gastroc Nemius, the huge calf muscle of Left Leg.

When the Inspector arrives at the great muscle, it's clear it has
been working overtime. The muscle bundles that make Left Leg
run are tired. They aren't pulling so hard. There isn't enough oxygen for efficient burning of fuel. Lactic acid waste is piling up. The
muscles feel as if they're on fire. They are not recovering well during the short rest periods. Nevertheless, the Inspector can't help
admire this powerful living machine as all the muscle cells work
together to move Left Leg quickly around the tennis court.

Inspector Bodyguard stands before Great Gastroc Nemius and
blows his whistle to get the attention of the muscle cell citizens.

"Muscle cells of Great Gastroc Nemius, I understand your situation. You don't have enough oxygen. You don't have enough water. But mostly, you don't have enough salt. I want you to know that it's okay with me if you go on strike."

"If we do, Inspector," says a spokesmuscle cell, "Brain will feel pain."

"It's time Brain felt pain," says the Inspector firmly. "Brain, with a mind of its own, is causing all of us to suffer. Let the strike begin!"

With a groan, the muscle cell citizens contract for a last time. They clench their jaws and hold fast in a rigid band. The entire Great Gastroc Nemius becomes knotted and solid. Normally, the muscle cell citizens relax as they take in salt after contracting. But now there is a shortage of water and salt. They can't relax, no matter how much they might want to. It's too bad, but the magnificent living machine has been brought to its knees.

The Land of U jolts to a stop. The Inspector can hear him yell with pain, "Owww! I've got a cramp."

"How long have you been out here, kid?" asks the tennis pro.

"About six hours" answers the Land of U.

"Have you been drinking anything?"

"No. I didn't want to stop playing."

"Don't you know how important it is to keep taking in fluids when you're active in weather like this. Come with me. I've got just the drink to replace both water and salt."

In a few minutes, Inspector Bodyguard hears the welcome slurping noises as Mouth Terminal receives its fluid. The Land of U is drinking a special concoction made for athletes that helps restore the body's balance of water and salt. The Inspector watches as the muscle cells slowly relax and the cramp starts easing up.

He heaves a sigh of relief. The dangerous, hot, dry spell is over. The Land of U will rest and recover. Soon all will be well again. Perhaps Brain has learned a lesson so that it won't happen again. The Keeper of the Health can only hope.

As the Land of U cools down in an air-conditioned room, Lipskin Passage curves into a smile. Brain's Memory Movies are replaying a forehand crosscourt winner against the club pro. It seems as if another lesson has also been learned today.

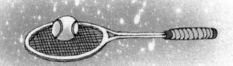

HOW———————— YOUR BODY DEALS WITH OVERHEATING

Heat is always being produced in your body. Some of the energy stored in food is released by living cells as heat. Muscular activity also produces heat. When surrounding temperatures are around 75 degrees, you feel most comfortable. This is because heat from your body is escaping into the surroundings at a rate equal to its replacement by normal activity.

If you exercise strenuously in 75 degree weather, you feel quite warm. Your body is now producing heat faster than the heat can escape into the surroundings. When the temperature of your surroundings is close to your normal body temperature, even without strenuous activity, heat does not move so quickly into the air. These are times when your body has to cool you off. To maintain normal body temperature of 98.6 degrees, your body must be able to get rid of extra heat.

Heat is energy that moves from areas of higher temperatures to areas of lower temperatures. The skin is where the body gets rid of extra heat and sends it to the surroundings. It does this by cooling the blood. Here's how.

The *hypothalamus* receives a message that there is too much heat in the body. When the weather is hot, this message comes from nerves on the skin. The hypothalamus activates the sympathetic nervous system. One of the results is a contraction of tiny muscles that squeeze the *sweat glands*. A sweat gland is a coiled tube located in the dermis. It is very tiny. You can see it only with a microscope. But if you could unravel it, the tube would be four feet long! Each sweat gland removes water and salt and certain wastes from the blood of nearby capillaries. The drop of sweat shoots up to the surface of the skin when the muscle squeezes. The sweat on your skin can now evaporate. Evaporation requires heat. Evaporating sweat uses heat from your skin, and in this way cools your skin and the underlying blood.

At the same time, the sympathetic nervous system makes the blood vessels near the skin open wider. This allows more blood to be circulated near the cooling surface. It also makes the skin appear flushed. A rosy appearance is typical of overheating.

You have two million sweat glands on your body. Each gland squirts out a drop of sweat every nine seconds or so. If you play tennis on a very hot day, your sweat glands can produce six times your normal amount of sweat, more than a gallon over several hours. If you lose too much water, you can create a dangerous condition. So the body takes steps to conserve water while it produces still more sweat to cool you off.

As blood is directed toward the skin, there is less blood for your digestive tract. If you have recently eaten, food may not be digested properly, giving you a feeling of an upset stomach. The hypothalamus also directs a very important nearby gland, the *pituitary*, to secrete a hormone that makes the kidneys reabsorb water from the blood. Normally, this water would be excreted in your urine. But the pituitary's hormone makes the urine more concentrated, keeping the extra water in your body to be available for sweat. The hormone also makes your mouth dry because less saliva is produced. A dry mouth makes you thirsty so that you drink to replace lost water.

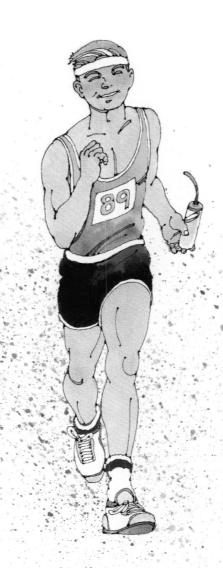

If you don't replace lost water and salt, and you continue to stay active in the sun, you are in danger of heat exhaustion. You may feel slightly dizzy and light-headed. You are tired and may have a headache. You may get muscle cramps, caused by overworking muscles that have lost salt through sweating. To treat heat exhaustion, you should give in to these feelings. It is best to stop your activities, rest in a cool, dry place and drink fluids. Lots of water and a few potato chips at dinner replace both water and salt lost by heavy sweating.

Continued activity after heat exhaustion sets in can put a person in danger of heat stroke. This is a truly life-threatening state. Sweating stops. The temperature of the body's core starts rising and the victim feels quite feverish. If core temperature goes above 106 degrees Fahrenheit, there is a danger of brain damage. The pulse pounds, and the victim may pass out. At first the skin is flushed, but it can become ashen and blue. Heat stroke is a medical emergency. It is important to get help fast because minutes count. Body temperature should be lowered as quickly as possible by putting the victim in cold (not ice) water or sponging the skin with cold water and fanning it dry. When the temperature gets down to 102 degrees, the person should be covered with a blanket to prevent a chill. Victims of heat stroke should be treated in a hospital for several days.

Experienced runners in marathons understand the importance of drinking water during a race. Before a race, runners will drink fluids for an hour or so. During the race they will take advantage of all the water stops along the course. Experienced runners have also had the benefit of good training programs. Their bodies can take the stress of performance in hot weather and they also know their own bodies.

Your body can protect you against rising temperatures only up to a point. You must do your part by taking extra fluids in hot weather and paying attention to the way you feel. Feeling tired and uncomfortable in hot weather is your body's way of telling you to take it easy. It's a message that should not fall on deaf ears.

8:

A PLUMBING FOULUP

"I'll have a steak, medium rare, a salad, French fries and a glass of chocolate milk." Inspector Bodyguard hears the Land of U giving his order at a restaurant. The nation's father is taking him and a friend out to lunch. "Good," thinks the Inspector, "Papilla Taste Bud and his friends will be happy. So will the cells down in Belly Bag Waiting Room. They won't need me. Let's see, what will I do today? I think I'll visit the citizens of Trachea Parkway and Bronchi Avenue. Just to make sure that oxygen imports keep getting through."

Trachea Parkway and Bronchi Avenue are main highways for the Air Import System that keep Red Cell Truckers supplied with the oxygen they bring to the rest of the Land of U.

"Mmmm. What's the best route to get there?" The Inspector consults his maps. "I think I'll take the Blood Buggy to Air Sac Lane. I can park there and then travel by foot up through Left Bronchi Avenue to Trachea Parkway."

By going this route, the Inspector knows that he will be walking in

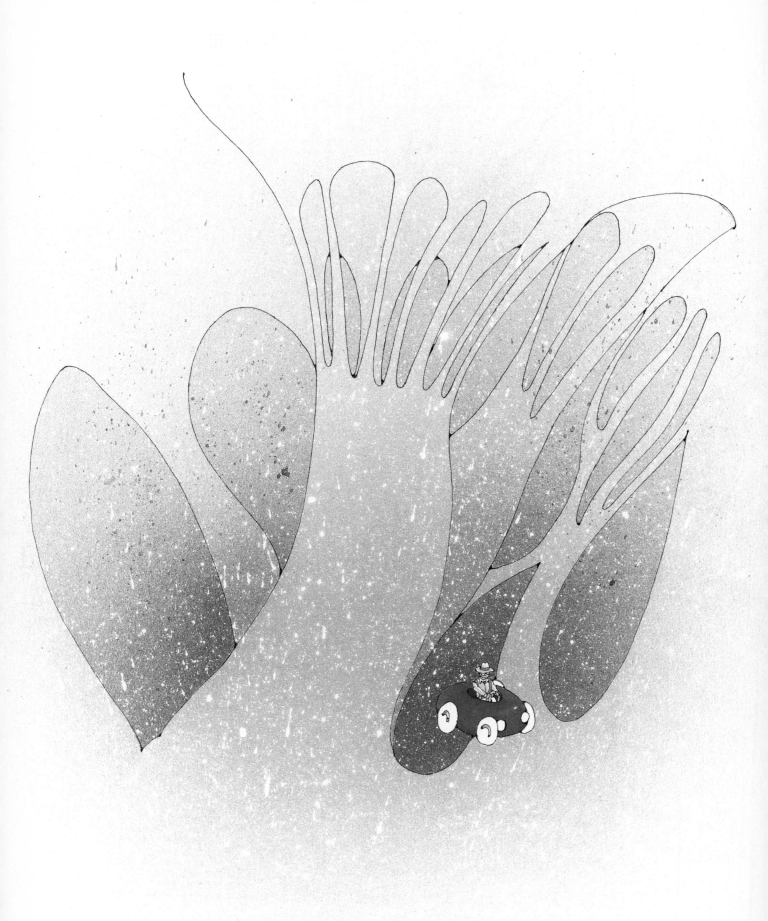

the same direction as the waving of the Living Hair Cells that line the highways. The Living Hair Cells have the job of beating out dust and other pollutants that come in from the Great Beyond with every imported breath of the great nation. The living hair cells wave together to sweep the stuff back out where it comes from. Walking in from Sinus Hill, along with the imported air, is like swimming upstream. Why should the Inspector trudge against the flow, when he can walk with it? And when it comes to traveling along the Air Passages, there's still the problem of wind resistance. No matter which way the Inspector moves, half the time the wind is at his back and half the time it's blowing in his face. A trip through Air Import System is alway interesting.

The Inspector relaxes in his Blood Buggy on his trip down from his office in Cortex Central. He has chosen to travel the blue blood route and admires the valves that flatten against the walls of the veins as he passes. "I think I'll take the Vena Cava through the heart and get to the left lung through the Pulmonary Artery. I'll arrive with the incoming Red Cell Truckers, who are exchanging carbon dioxide waste for a load of oxygen."

The sound of the heart valves opening and closing grows louder as the Inspector draws near the Great Pump of the Red River. Incredible structure! Inspector Bodyguard's heart swells with pride as he watches the perfect performance of the powerful muscle. Two loud "lub-dubs" and the Inspector is through the heart and on his way to the lungs.

He knows he is close to Air Sac Lane as the Red River gets smaller and smaller. Soon he is in a tiny capillary just wide enough to let one Red Cell Trucker through at a time. It's also a tight squeeze for the Blood Buggy. Inspector Bodyguard watches a truck pick up a load of oxygen. As soon as the oxygen is on board the Trucker changes from blue to red. With a smile of satisfaction, the Inspector squeezes through the capillary wall into the lacy structure of Air Sac Lane. The howl of the wind sings along with the Air Sac Lane cells.

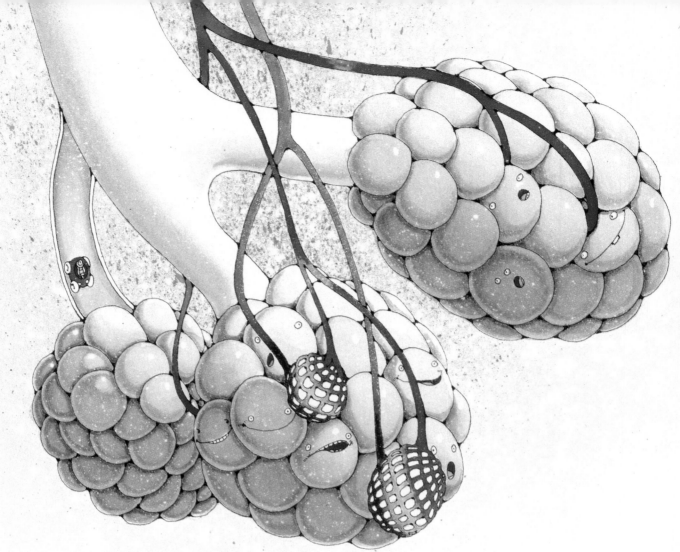

Oxygen! Oh Oxygen!
The gas that we adore.
If we don't get our quota,
U would pass out on the floor.

Oxygen! Oh Oxygen!
Without it, blood is blue.
For every molecule that we take,
We trade one of C-0-two.

Oxygen! Oh Oxygen!
Without it all would die.
But there's no chance that we'll run short,
There's plenty in the sky.

Oxygen! Oh Oxygen!
We love it! Yes, we do!
So we keep those trade winds blowing,
Exchanging old, used gas for new.

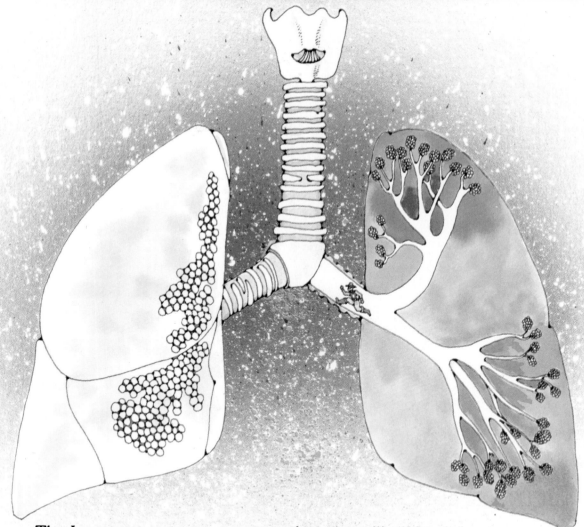

The Inspector waves to a group of air sac cells. "How's business on the air exchange, today?"

"Can't complain, Inspector. We get our share," answers an air sac cell.

"Good. Well, if you don't mind, I think I'll hike on up through the Air Import System."

"Go right ahead, Inspector. The weather should be okay. We don't see any activity that would cause the wind speed to pick up." The air sac cell feels a little tickle as an oxygen molecule passes through him to a waiting Red Cell Trucker.

Inspector Bodyguard enthusiastically begins his hike. The tiny Air Sac Lane where he begins his trek soon joins with others to form a much larger bronchiole street. The bronchiole streets come together to form the large Left Bronchi Avenue. The Inspector feels short bursts of air at his back as he turns up Trachea Parkway. The Land of U is laughing and the sound echoes all around him.

Inspector Bodyguard can also hear the sound of chewing. From the slow deliberate "chomp, chomp" he knows that the steak is not very tender. From the Great Beyond he hears a boy's voice. The friend of the Land of U is telling a joke. There is no way for the Inspector to know that he is in a potentially very dangerous situation.

As the friend finishes the punch line, a powerful blast of air rushes by the Inspector, knocking him off his feet. A huge "guffaw" explodes from the voice box of the Land of U. "That must have been some joke," thinks the Inspector as he pulls himself upright with the help of a living hair cell. Suddenly there is a piece of steak at his feet.

"Hey," yells a living hair cell, "this doesn't belong here. Steak is a far cry from air!"

"Let's beat it out of here," cries another.

"We can't. It's too heavy!" moans a third. Panic is entering his voice.

The air sac cells are crying from deep in the lungs.

"What's happened to our oxygen? We need oxygen! We need oxygen!"

This is indeed a serious state. The steak must be removed before it cuts off the oxygen supply to the lungs!

"Don't tell me about it," the Inspector says to the cells of Trachea Parkway. "Get the message on Vagus Nerve Circuit to Major Medulla. This is his kind of problem."

Major Medulla is the master of reflex action. He always acts correctly without thinking.

Inspector Bodyguard doesn't have to wait long for the response. Within half a second he feels the strong wind in his face. This means that Great Diaphragm, the sheet of muscle that runs under the lungs from the ribs to the back, has moved down. This makes the chest cavity larger and lowers the air pressure in the lungs. Air rushes in, as if the lungs are a vacuum cleaner.

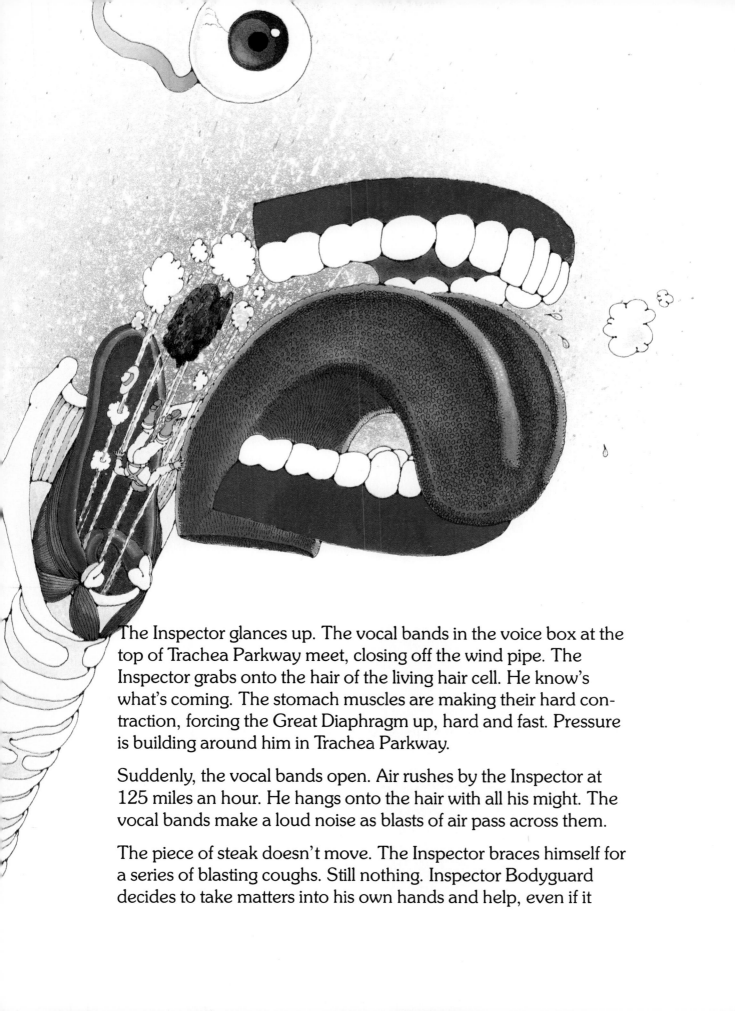

The Inspector glances up. The vocal bands in the voice box at the top of Trachea Parkway meet, closing off the wind pipe. The Inspector grabs onto the hair of the living hair cell. He know's what's coming. The stomach muscles are making their hard contraction, forcing the Great Diaphragm up, hard and fast. Pressure is building around him in Trachea Parkway.

Suddenly, the vocal bands open. Air rushes by the Inspector at 125 miles an hour. He hangs onto the hair with all his might. The vocal bands make a loud noise as blasts of air pass across them.

The piece of steak doesn't move. The Inspector braces himself for a series of blasting coughs. Still nothing. Inspector Bodyguard decides to take matters into his own hands and help, even if it

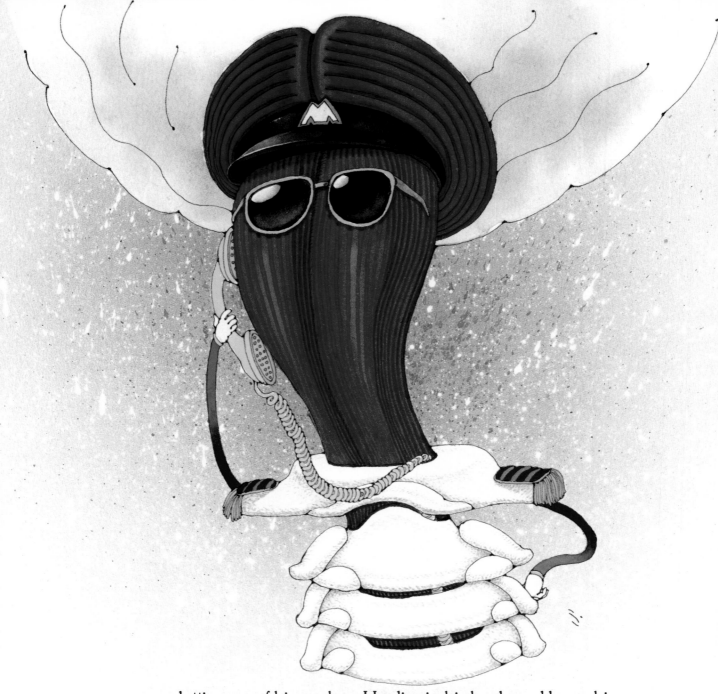

means letting go of his anchor. He digs in his heels and leans his shoulder against the steak. He begins to push as the vocal bands close above him.

The powerful rush of air blasts both the Inspector and the piece of steak up through Epiglottis Safety Valve to the back of Tongue Receiving Station. The coughing stops. But the Inspector has to grab onto a taste bud as a tidal wave of water passes over him in the other direction back to Throat Elevator. After the swallow and the reopening of the Epiglottis Safety Valve, he can hear the cheering of the cell citizens of Trachea Parkway.

"Whew! That was a scare!" The Inspector calls Major Medulla on the Axon Messenger Service.

"That was a close one, Major. Congratulations on having your circuits in order."

"Appreciate the call, Inspector. Sure was a mix-up down there. Epiglottis Safety Valve didn't close and keep out the food. That's the danger of eating and talking and laughing at the same time. Wires get crossed and the pipes are mixed up."

"Yes, well, these things happen. Wouldn't want the Land of U to stop laughing. Anyhow, it's our job to protect the Land of U in just this kind of situation. At least this time we solved the problem ourselves and didn't need help from the Great Beyond. Thanks again, Major."

The Inspector turns and quietly slips through Epiglottis Safety Valve, back to Trachea Parkway. He has come further than he had planned and it will be a long hike, walking against the beating of the living hair cells, back to his Blood Buggy.

"Oh well," he shrugs, "might as well enjoy the gentle breezes and fine weather. It's also a good chance to get a breath of fresh air."

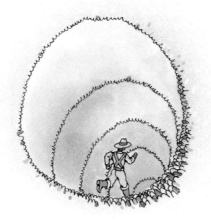

HOW
YOUR COUGH PROTECTS
YOU

Energy for living comes from a chemical reaction between food and oxygen. A fire is the release of heat and light energy as a fuel combines rapidly with oxygen. The end products of a fire are carbon dioxide and water. In your body, a fuel (food) also combines with oxygen to produce carbon dioxide and water. Only the reaction does not release the energy all at once, as in a fire. Instead, the combination of fuel with oxygen is broken down into many steps. Each step is carefully controlled by enzymes in all your cells. Controlled release makes the energy available for movement, nerve impulses, growth, repair, and all the other things cells must do to keep you alive. Without oxygen, most of these activities quickly come to a halt. Death follows almost immediately. So it's no surprise that the body has an efficient system for getting oxygen and that it also has ways to protect this system.

Air comes into the lungs as your *diaphragm* moves downward. The diaphragm is a sheetlike muscle that separates your chest from your abdomen. When it moves down, it makes the chest cavity larger. The pressure on the outside of the lungs becomes lower than air pressure in the atmosphere. Air rushes into the lungs to fill this partial vacuum.

Incoming air moves to fill all the spaces in the lungs. The air passages are like a tree, becoming more and more divided. The tiniest branches are the *air sacs* or *alveoli*. The walls of the air sacs are one cell thick. Capillaries, with walls also one cell thick, are right next to the alveoli walls. Red blood cells are in the capillaries ready to exchange the waste gas, carbon dioxide, for the incoming gas, oxygen. Carbon dioxide-carrying red cells are bluish in color. After the gas exchange, they become bright red.

Air gets to the lungs through a tube called the *trachea*, or windpipe, which lies along side the esophagus. The walls of the trachea are held in an open circle by rings of *cartilage*, stiff but flexible material you also find at the end of your nose. The top of the trachea is the voice box. Both the esophagus and the voice box open at the back of the throat. It is of the utmost importance to keep food out of the trachea so that nothing blocks incoming air. So when you swallow, the *epiglottis*, a flap of cartilage at the top of the voice box, lowers over the opening. Food passes over the closed epiglottis, keeping it out of the windpipe.

When you laugh, your epiglottis is open. Air is moving out of your lungs, over your vocal cords in your voice box. If you have food in your mouth when you laugh, there is always the danger that a morsel can slip through the open epiglottis into the trachea. A large morsel of food can block the windpipe, causing you to choke.

The defense against choking is the cough *reflex*. A reflex is an automatic response you don't have to think about. Here's how the cough reflex works.

An irritating substance in the trachea triggers a nerve ending that sends an impulse along the large *vagus* nerve. The impulse travels up the vagus nerve to the breathing center in the *medulla*, the enlarged end of the spinal chord that forms the base of the brain. Nerves from the medulla, returning to the muscles of the diaphragm which control breathing, cause the diaphragm to move

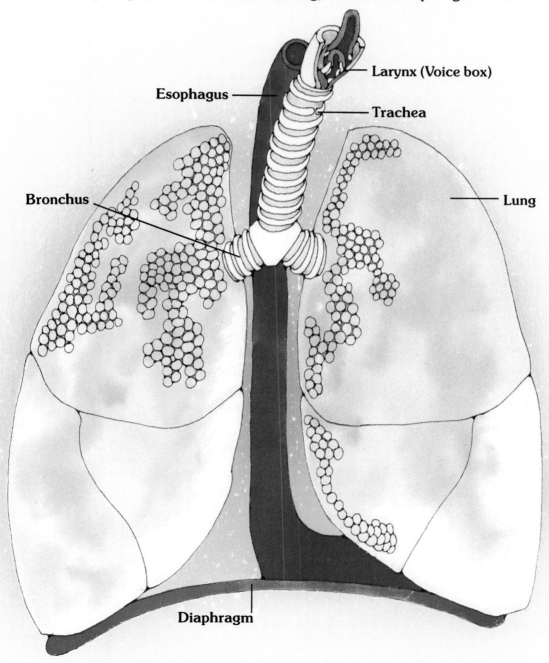

Esophagus

Larynx (Voice box)

Trachea

Bronchus

Lung

Diaphragm

down. As a result, air is inhaled into the lungs. The epiglottis and the vocal chords close as the diaphragm moves up. This increases the pressure of the trapped air, suddenly pushing the vocal bands and the epiglottis open. Air rushes out, hopefully carrying the irritating materials with it.

If a person can cough or talk when choking, you know that the trachea is only partially blocked. Air can still be inhaled. There are times when the trachea is completely blocked. The choking person cannot breathe at all. His or her hand goes automatically to the throat.

A simple move, called the *Heimlich maneuver*, can save the life of a choking person. The purpose of the Heimlich maneuver is to give a sharp squeeze to the diaphragm, increasing the force of the air coming out of the lungs. If it is given properly, the expelled air has enough force to dislodge the obstacle. You can learn the Heimlich maneuver in a first aid course. It is not hard to do. A four-year-old who saw it on TV used it to save the life of his two-year-old brother, who was choking on a toy.

When you are sick, extra mucus forms in your air passages. Coughing moves the mucus out of the trachea into the throat where you can swallow it, or spit it out.

9:

THE CHICKENPOX WAR

Inspector Bodyguard always stops by Sinus Hill on his daily patrol of the Land of U. Sinus Hill is a popular target of all kinds of germs floating around in the air of the Great Beyond. Most of the time, germs that come in with inhaled air never get a foothold among the cell citizens of the Air Import System. When the cell citizens are happy and healthy, enemies of the Land of U don't stand a chance. Inspector Bodyguard's visits keep up the good spirits. It works both ways. When his cells are happy, he is, too.

So, in his usual cheerful way, Inspector Bodyguard gives Sinus Hill citizens a pat on the back. This particular early spring day is no different from any other. When he arrives, he blows his whistle three times and says, "My friends of Sinus Hill, keep beating out the dust and germs that come your way. Keep that mucus flowing. Keep those passages free and clear. Keep up all your good work. I thank you on behalf of all the cell citizens of the Land of U."

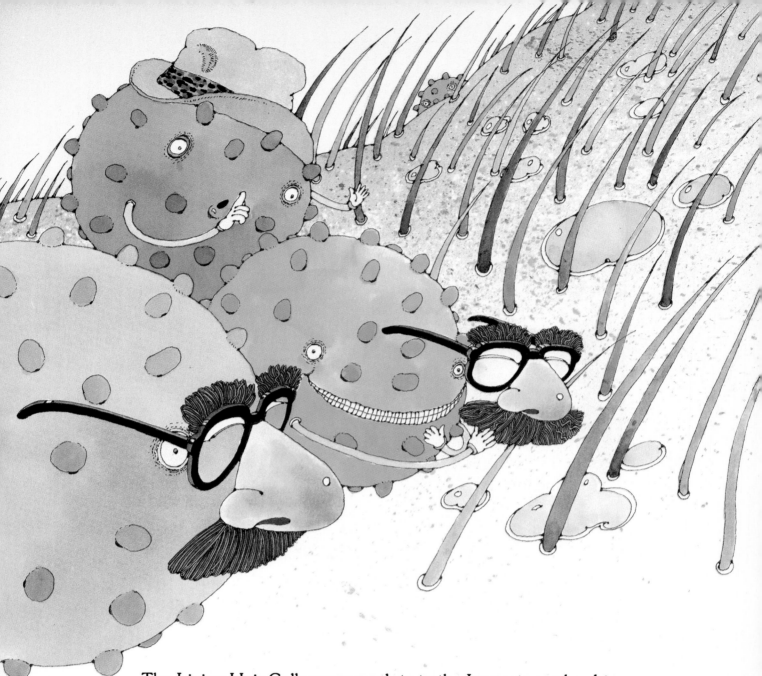

The Living Hair Cells wave a salute to the Inspector as he drives off in his Blood Buggy. At that very moment no one realizes that Sinus Hill is being invaded by a particularly sneaky enemy, thousands of almost invisible chickenpox viruses. There is something to be said for an army of cold or flu viruses, who make themselves known to the citizens of Sinus Hill almost as soon as they land. These enemies can then be dealt with immediately. You know what you're fighting. But the chickenpox viruses have a different attack plan.

Like the cold viruses, they travel in from the Great Beyond in glittering water droplets. Just before entering Nose Cavern, a troop of chickenpox viruses glances longingly at Skin Frontier.

"Boy, oh boy! Look at that delicious territory. Are we going to have fun marking that up!" gloats one of the immature pox troopers.

"We're not ready for that yet, so cool it and keep quiet." says the Pox Group Leader. "We've got two weeks to get strong and organized once we land. We don't start marking up Skin Frontier until I say so. Meantime, we'll lie low and increase our numbers."

Silently the pox troopers land on Sinus Hill and disappear among the cell citizens. A few cells may have some suspicions that something is afoot, but they don't know enough to say anything. The pox troopers thrive in the warm, moist, fertile atmosphere of the Air Import System. Other pox trooper groups are quietly doing their thing in the Small Gut Tunnel. The Land of U and the Inspector go about their daily business, completely ignorant of the army in their midst, an army that is gaining strength, day by day. The pox troopers smile knowingly at each other each time the Inspector visits Sinus Hill and congratulates the cell citizens there for doing a fine job. They know their time will come.

Two weeks, almost to the minute, after they landed on Sinus Hill, the attack readiness signal travels among the chickenpox troops. A thrill of excitement runs through them. It's time! Let the fun begin! They shake loose from their little nests among the citizens of Sinus Hill and Small Gut Tunnel. A few of them ride out in droplets on air exhaled from Nose Cavern into the Great Beyond, hoping to find other Human Bodies to attack. But most of them—and by now there are millions—slip quietly into the Red River.

Their arrival in the bloodstream does not go unnoticed.

"Halt! Who goes there, friend or foe?" demands a sentry white cell.

"None of your business. Out of my way, paleface. I'm going to make my mark on your land!" The chickenpox trooper pushes past the white cell.

"I'd better release my Pyrogen Firestarter. We're up against an unknown enemy. At least this will give them something to think about." The sentry cell squeezes a little of the chemical into the Red River.

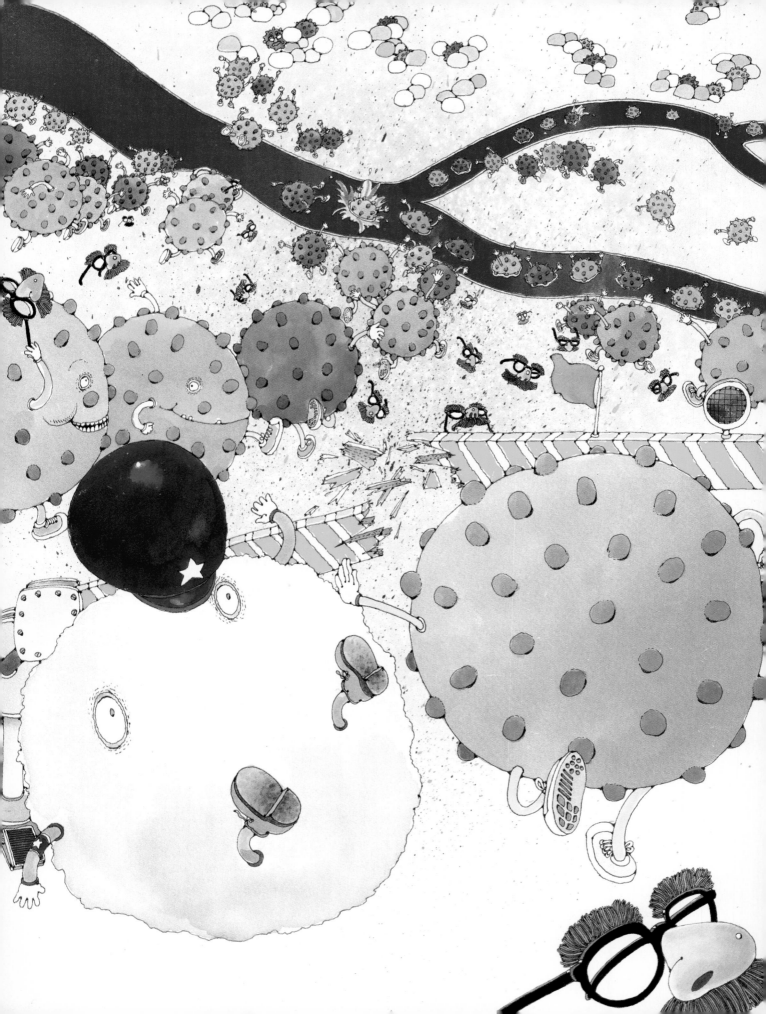

The Pyrogen Firestarter travels through the bloodstream with the firestarters from other sentry cells. In a short time, it reaches a part of Brain Command Post right behind the eyes. The nerves fire. Almost instantly the red alert goes off in the Hypothalamus Computer Base. At the same time, Inspector Bodyguard gets the message in his office. He doesn't waste any time getting Chief Underbrain of HCB on the wire.

"What have we got, Chief? A Firestarter Alert Condition?"

"Right, Inspector. I'm about to raise the thermostat and give U fever."

"That's pretty drastic action. You know that it will affect the entire nation. Brain isn't going to like it. We're not going to be able to do our usual activities or go to school. But if the red alert is on, we have no choice. Throw the switch, Chief. I'm on my way to check out the enemy."

The Inspector hangs up on Chief Underbrain and purposefully puts in a call to Captain Blast, head of the Germbusters. The Captain must have been expecting the call because he is instantly on the wire.

"Captain Blast, here, Inspector. We've got problems?"

"Chief Underbrain reports a Firestarter Alert Condition. Obviously we've been invaded. Can't understand it. I've visited Sinus Hill every day and there hasn't been a sign." The Inspector's voice was puzzled. It was not like him to be puzzled long.

"My sentries report an invasion of viruses. They seem to be heading for Skin Frontier. My guess is that that's where the battle will take place," says Captain Blast.

"You'd better join me in the Blood Buggy, Captain. Let's head for Skin Frontier and keep our eyes open for clues as we go.

By the time Inspector Bodyguard and Captain Blast begin their trip to the battlefield, the fever started by Chief Underbrain is well underway. At first the Land of U reacts the way he reacted to the chill last summer from swimming in cold water too long. Blood vessels near Skin Frontier grow smaller, keeping the blood near

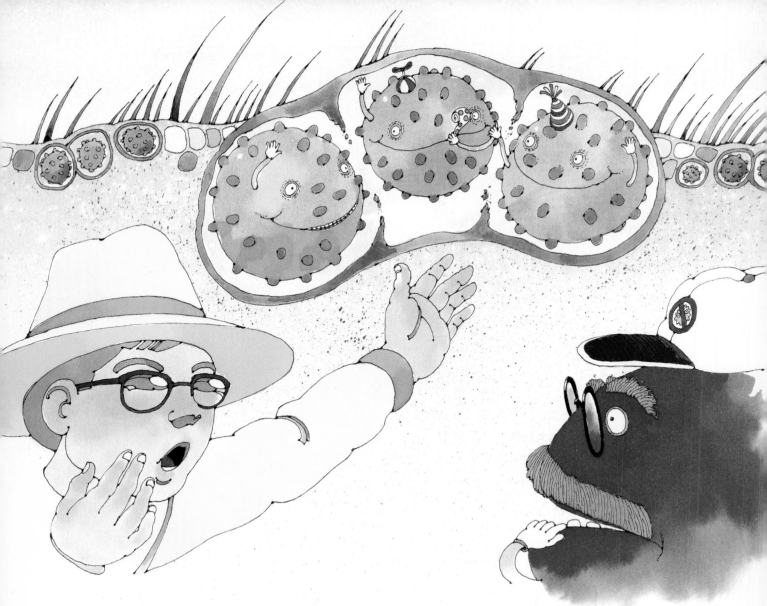

the heartland, where it's warmer. The Hairy Pilis pull their weight and make goose bumps on Skin Frontier. Chill after chill passes through the nation. Brain is complaining. Whimpering sounds come from the voice box. The Inspector feels the Land of U lie down. He knows that many blankets are being used to make him feel warm.

Then the shivering begins. Bundles of muscle cells receive the message to start contracting. Brain cannot control the motion. There is a loud clattering from Mouth Receiving Station as the jaw muscles cause the back teeth to bang together. As expected, the increased muscle activity generates heat. The temperature of the entire nation rises. Inspector Bodyguard knows that now is not the time to lower it. He takes out his handkerchief and mops his brow.

"Hopefully, things will now get a bit hot for our enemy, Captain," comments the Inspector.

"Well, increased temperatures do make all the cell citizens work faster, and some of our enemies are slowed down. In any case, it is a clear message that the Land of U is working on the problem," says Captain Blast.

As the blood Buggy nears Skin Frontier, they can hear the war whoops of the pox troops. The battle is in full swing. The pox troops are singing their spirited battle hymn:

Charge forward, fellow viruses!
Invade a cell or two
Then let us join together
And make a chickenpox on U.

Let cells try to fight us
No matter what they do
Red spots of our graffiti
Make a chickenpox on U.

We make the top skin separate
And fill the space with goo,
Small, itchy blisters are a stage
Of chickenpox on U.

And when the blisters break, my
    friend,
You think perhaps we're through
But no. Now there is a scab
For each chickenpox on U.

Scratch a scab so it comes off
Baring skin that's raw and new,
A scar forever marks the spot
Of that chickenpox on U.

To the battle, fellow viruses!
We're more noteworthy than flu
They just make U feel bad,
We make our chickenpox on U.

Inspector Bodyguard and Captain Blast watch with horrified eyes as the chickenpox troops advance with war whoops and battle cries. The target of each trooper is a Prickle Cell of Skin Frontier. In no time, a virus passes through the cell membrane and is living inside the cell. And then a strange thing begins to happen. The cell membranes of infected cells next to each other dissolve. The insides of the cells run together, creating a monstrous giant cell. Pox troopers inside this giant cell greet each other as if they haven't seen each other in weeks.

The Inspector can hear the cries of the injured Prickle Cells.

"No, please…I don't want to lose my identity."

"I know I'm supposed to love my neighbor…I just don't want to blend with him."

"There are worse ways to go. At least we'll have company in our misery."

Inspector Bodyguard blows his whistle for attention. "Release your liquid warning! Release histamine!" he yells.

Gasping and crying, the wounded cells respond to their leader's command.

"That will bring in more of my bloody army," observes Captain Blast. Sure enough, the blood rushes to the scene of the battle, causing small red pimples to form on the surface of Skin Frontier wherever cells have been invaded.

"Better activate the Lymphocyte Antibody Division for this job, Blast. I have a hunch that we're only going to get rid of these poxmakers with our ultimate weapon."

"I'm ahead of you, Inspector. They're already tooling up. But I'm afraid we're not going to solve this battle quickly."

"We'll let it run its course, Blast. Let's just hope there are no complications. Wait! Suffering synapses! What's happening now?"

The Inspector and the Captain feel heavy pressure pass over them. They are squeezed together and then released, not once but three times.

"I've got to see what's happening," says the Inspector. He quickly

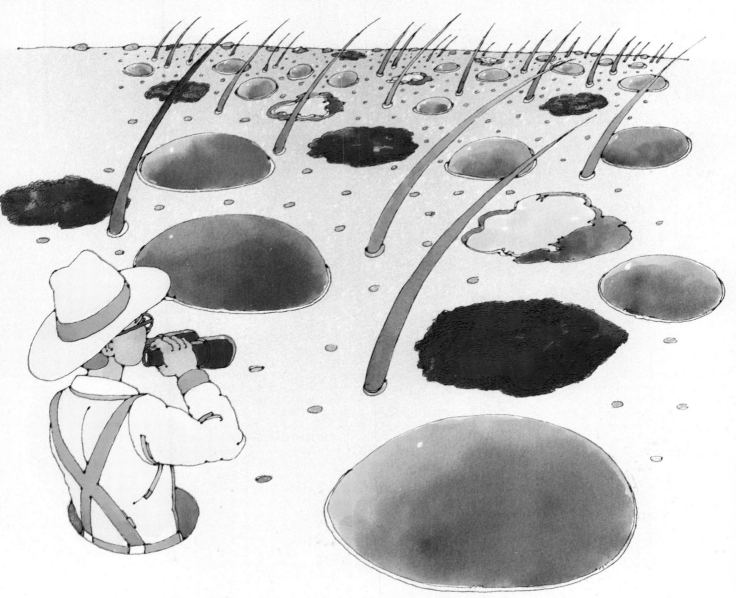

moves to a nearby sweat gland and climbs up its tube to a pore on the surface of Skin Frontier. Because of the fever, there was no sweat in the way. As the Inspector sticks out his head, an amazing sight greets his eyes. As far as he can see, Skin Frontier is dotted with red pimples. Obviously, they are creating a problem for the Land of U, because Hands' Ends are busy scratching. That was the pressure the two guardians had felt. The Inspector quickly ducks back inside the pore as the great Right Hand's End presses over him.

Inspector Bodyguard reports on the problem to his Captain. "These tiny sores caused by the enemy are not bad enough to make the free nerve endings send a pain message. But they do tickle them enough to send an itch message. And Hands' Ends are scratching away."

"There's nothing we can do about that. Let's hope there's some lotion or other medicine that can be applied from the Great Beyond. It's our job to get rid of the enemy," replies Captain Blast.

The pimple they are watching is changing. The giant cell formed by the viruses is separating from the top layer of dead skin cells. The space is filling with the clear fluid. When the Inspector checks the surface, he sees many of the red pimples are now clear, domed hills filled with fluid.

The war is already in its fourth day and the Antibody Division of the White Cell Civil Defense is starting to have an effect. Specially made antibodies are killing the viruses one on one. The bodies of dead viruses are found floating in the liquid of the poxes. The Big Macro Germ Eating Units are eating up the debris.

By the beginning of the second week, many of the poxes have broken open, spilling their fluid. But Captain Blast's platelets are right there making scabs. The fever has disappeared. The temperature is normal.

"We're on the home stretch, Inspector," says Captain Blast as he checks the structural strength of a scab.

"Let's just hope that itching doesn't make Hands' Ends scratch off a scab. Then we'll have to deal with those awful bacteria that cause infection. Skin Frontier will never recover perfectly. The repair will always show as a scar." The Inspector looks tired. A war like this keeps him busier than usual.

In the week that follows, the Inspector and Captain Blast oversee the winning battles between antibodies and the pox troopers. The Land of U has normal activities, although he remains at home. No school for U until the last pox has scabbed over.

Finally, the Inspector and the Captain can claim victory.

"You know the best thing about this war, Captain?" asks the Inspector as they watch the final stages of the cleanup and repair.

"What's that Inspector?"

"We'll never have to deal with those viruses again. The antibodies we made to fight them will be with us for life."

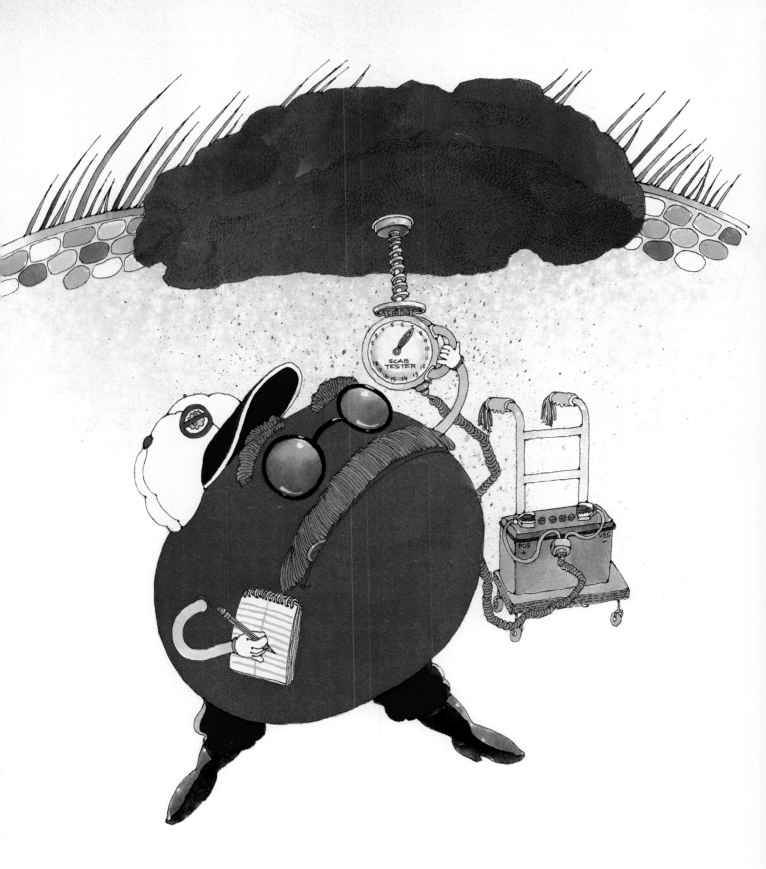

The Inspector turns to the citizens of Skin Frontier, who are watching the remains of the enemy disappear in the cleanup. He blows his whistle. "You hear that, my friends? Never again! We are finished with the poxes. We are immune to their warfare!"

The Inspector and the Captain make V-for-victory signs with their fingers as the citizens of Skin Frontier give a resounding cheer.

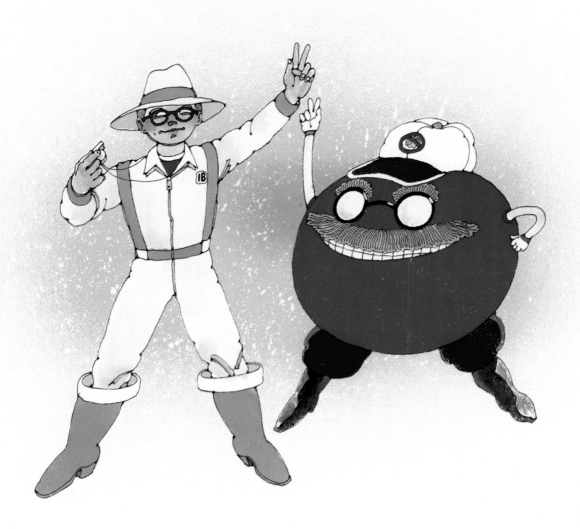

HOW

YOUR BODY FIGHTS CHICKENPOX

Chickenpox is a very contagious disease that most people get during child-hood. It is caused by a virus that enters the body through the air. After a person has been exposed to the virus, there is an incubation period of thirteen to seventeen days before the disease appears. During the incubation period, the person doesn't feel sick at all.

Scientists aren't sure exactly what the virus does during the incubation period. They think the viruses multiply in the respiratory system and in the intestines. At the end of the incubation period, they move to the skin through the blood stream.

The first symptoms of chickenpox are a fever and a feeling of illness. You may have a headache. A fever is the body's response to an infection. Certain white blood cells release a chemical called *endogenous pyrogen* into the blood-stream. When the endogenous pyrogens reach a part of the brain behind the eyes, the nerves send messages to the hypothalamus and the body's thermo-stat is set higher. The fever begins.

The first signs of a fever are chills and feeling cold. You want to get warm and can't seem to get enough blankets on you. Then shivering begins. It is the shiv-ering that actually raises your body temperature. Moving muscles generate heat. The uncontrolled muscle movement of shivering causes your tempera-ture to rise.

It is not fun to have a fever. For many years, people took drugs, like aspirin, that made a fever "break." When a fever breaks you have the opposite reac-tion to that of being chilled. Blood vessels near the skin open wide. Your skin becomes flushed as more blood circulates near the surface, and you sweat. The sweating cools you off and thus brings down your fever. If you don't take any drugs, the breaking of a fever is a sign that you are on the mend.

Recently, doctors have concluded that a fever is an important defense against infection. All the chemical reactions involved in the life processes happen faster when you are warm. This may give the cells fighting the disease an ad-vantage, because some infecting germs may not function as well when the temperature is high. So doctors may recommend that you let a fever run its course, rather than take drugs to lower it. Of course, if the fever is very high—

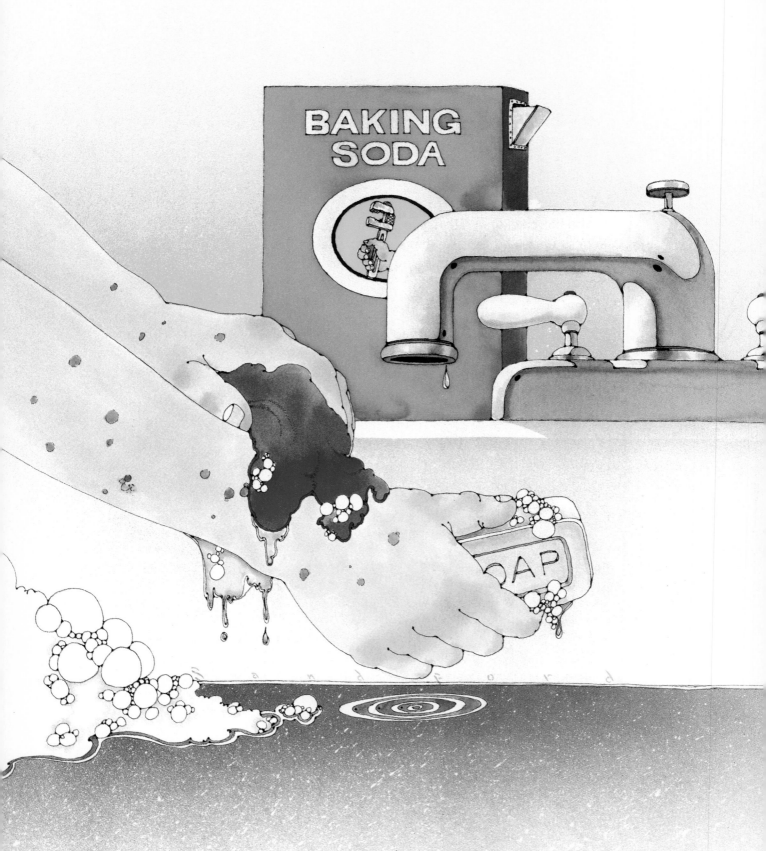

perhaps 105 degrees Fahrenheit—or if it runs for more than a few days, treatment may be suggested. In any case, you should always drink a lot of liquids if you have a fever, because the body will lose fluid when the fever breaks.

A day or two after the first feelings of illness, the chickenpox rash starts breaking out. New crops of spots develop over the body for about four days. At first the rash is made up of tiny, red, itchy spots. These spots change in a day or two to tiny, dome-shaped blisters. Then the blisters break and the spots scab over. If the scabs are allowed to remain on the skin until they fall off naturally, there are no scars. The biggest danger of chickenpox is infection that may develop in the poxes if the scab is scratched off before the underlying skin has healed.

A person who has chickenpox can give it to others from the day before the first signs of illness until all the poxes have scabs. The antibodies that the body makes against the chickenpox virus stay in the bloodstream for life. This gives you permanent immunity against having chickenpox a second time.

In some people, however, the chickenpox virus lives quietly among the nerves near the spinal cord. Sometimes, many years later, the viruses attack the adult. Instead of getting a chickenpox rash all over the body, the viruses make a rash along a nerve, usually in the lower back. The disease is called "shingles" because there may be rows of rash along the nerves. Instead of itching, shingles is very painful.

Smallpox is a deadly virus disease that was one of the main causes of death in earlier centuries. People lucky enough to survive the disease had lifetime immunity against getting it again. But the rash left deep, ugly scars. About 200 years ago, Dr. Edward Jenner of England noticed that milkmaids who got cowpox, a very mild disease, never got smallpox. Dr. Jenner took the fluid from a cowpox blister on a milkmaid and injected it into the skin of a young boy. The young boy soon developed cowpox. A few months later, Dr. Jenner injected the boy with smallpox virus. The boy did not get the disease, and the world had its first example of developing immunity from a *vaccination*.

Vaccination against smallpox has virtually wiped the disease off the face of the earth. And today, vaccinations have given us protection against other diseases such as polio, mumps and measles. There is no readily available vaccine for chickenpox, however, although one is presently being developed.

GLOSSARY

Adrenalin—A hormone made by nerve endings and the adrenal medulla that causes the heart to beat faster and the lungs to breathe more deeply.

Adrenal medulla—The center of the gland located on top of each kidney. It secretes adrenalin to prepare the body for flight or fight when under stress.

Agglutination—The clumping reaction that occurs when two proteins of opposite shapes come together. When a microorganism and its antibody meet in the blood, agglutination takes place.

Air sacs (alveoli)—The tiny air cells of the lungs where oxygen is absorbed and carbon dioxide is eliminated.

Alpha waves—A pattern of electricity from the brain that occurs when the mind is at rest and able to function at its highest level.

Ameba—A one-celled animal that constantly changes its shape to move and to take in food.

Ameboid motion—Movement by cells that resembles the movement of amebas. White blood cells in the human body have ameboid motion.

Antibody—A protein substance made by the body to react with foreign material entering the body.

Antihistamine—A drug given to prevent the action of histamine released during an allergic attack. It's used to counter allergic reactions and to cut down on the swelling in a stuffy nose.

Appestat—The area of the hypothalamus that controls the appetite.

Arrector pili—A tiny muscle connected to the cells around a hair. When a person is cold or frightened, the arrector pili contracts, causing goose bumps.

Artery—A blood vessel that carries blood away from the heart.

ATP—The initials of a substance found in all cells that provides energy for all activities.

Autonomic nervous system—A part of the nervous system that controls involuntary activities such as gland secretions, the heartbeat, and reactions to emergencies.

Axon—A long, tubelike extension of a nerve cell that carries a nervous impulse from one place to another. Bundles of axons make up nerves.

Bacteria—One-celled microbes that must use an outside food supply in order to grow and reproduce. Bacteria may be beneficial or harmful to people.

Basal skin cells—The deepest cells of the epidermis. They are constantly dividing in two to replace older, worn out cells.

Bile—A thick, bitter secretion of the liver that helps break up fats in the small intestine so that they can be digested.

Blast—A young cell that hasn't yet fully developed.

Bronchi—The two main branches of the windpipe leading to a lung.

Bronchiole—A very small branch of a bronchus that ends in an air sac.

Capillary—The tiniest blood vessels that connect the ends of the smallest arteries with the smallest veins.

Cardiac—A word that is associated with the heart. The cardiac sphincter is a muscle closing off the upper end of the stomach, nearest to the heart.

Cartilage—A flexible, whitish material that protects the ends of bones. It is also found in the ears and the tip of the nose.

Chickenpox—A childhood disease caused by a virus and characterized by a body rash that starts out as red pimples, becomes tiny blisters, and ends up with scabs.

Chyme—A mixture of partly digested food and digestive juices found in the stomach and the beginning of the small intestine.

Cilia—Hairlike extensions of cells lining the air passages.

Cold-blooded—Describing animal life whose body temperature is the same as the surrounding temperature.

Contagious disease—Any disease that can be transmitted from one person to another, usually through the air.

Cortex—The outer layer of a structure. The cerebral cortex of the brain in man is more highly developed than in any other animal. The cerebral cortex is responsible for human intelligence.

Dermis—The underlying layer of skin containing the blood vessels and nerves.

Diaphragm—A thin, muscular wall that separates the chest cavity from the abdomen. It moves down so the lungs can inhale air and moves up to expel air from the lungs as we breathe.

Digestion—The process of breaking foods down, mechanically and chemically, so that they can be absorbed by the body.

Endogenous—Arising from within the body. *Exogenous* substances originate from outside the body.

Endogenous pyrogen—A substance that causes a fever, arising within the body.

Enzyme—A protein that controls chemical reactions in living things. Digestive enzymes break down food. Enzymes in cells regulate all the activities of cells.

Epidermis—The outer layer of the skin, composed partly of dead cells.

Epiglottis—The leaf-shaped flap that covers the opening to the voice box and trachea when swallowing.

Esophagus—A muscular tube that carries food from the back of the throat to the stomach.

Fever—A condition of body temperature above the normal 98.6 degrees Fahrenheit that is a reaction to an infection.

Fibrin—A white, hairlike protein that forms a network which is the "skeleton" of a blood clot.

Fibrinogen—A protein that is dissolved in blood plasma that becomes fibrin when acted upon by enzymes released during an injury to blood vessels.

Gamma globulin—A protein found in the blood that helps resist infections.

Ganglia—Groups of nerve cells that lie outside the spinal cord.

Gastrocnemius—The topmost muscle of the calf of the leg. It extends the foot and helps to bend the knee.

Goblet cells—Cells that makes mucus. They are found in the lining of the air passages and in the small intestine.

Heat exhaustion—Weakness, dizziness, nausea and headache in response to a long period in hot temperatures and loss of body fluids.

Heat stroke—A dangerous condition in which there is high body temperature, no sweating, fast pulse, and shallow breathing. It can result in death without proper medical treatment.

Heimlich maneuver—First aid for choking. It forces air out of the lungs by a sudden squeeze of the abdomen.

Hemophilia—A blood disease, inherited mostly by males, where the blood doesn't clot and bleeding can be uncontrolled.

Hemorrhage—Heavy, uncontrolled bleeding either outside or inside the body.

Histamine—A chemical given off during an allergic attack, or by injured cells, that causes blood vessels to expand.

Hormone—A chemical produced by a gland in one part of the body that travels through the blood and has an effect on another part of the body. Adrenalin is a hormone produced by the adrenal medulla that has an effect on the heart and lungs.

Host—The living thing that serves as nourishment to another living thing that invades it.

Hypothalamus—A small body under the center of the brain that controls a number of automatic body functions. These include the balance between salt and water, body temperature, and the balance between the sympathetic and parasympathetic divisions of the autonomic nervous system.

Immunity—Ability to resist a disease because previous exposure has caused the body to make antibodies.

Keratin—A tough protein that protects the skin and makes up hair and nails.

Lactic acid—A waste product of muscle activity that forms when there is a shortage of oxygen.

Liver—The largest organ of the body, located just under the diaphragm in the abdomen. It secretes bile, to aid digestion. It removes and stores sugar from the blood and manufactures a number of important body proteins, plus many other important jobs.

Lymph—A clear, colorless body fluid found in spaces between cells all over the body and in lymph vessels.

Lymph node—A rounded collection of many lymph vessels and white blood cells. White cells are produced in lymph nodes, and germs entering lymph nodes are prevented from entering the blood stream.

Lymphocyte—A type of white blood cell that is believed to remove certain poisonous wastes from the body.

Macrophages—Large amebalike white blood cells that "eat" germs at the site of infections.

Medulla—The inner or central part of an organ. The *medulla oblongata* is the enlarged part of the spinal cord where the spinal cord connects with the brain. It is responsible for controlling respiration and blood pressure, among other functions.

Molecule—The smallest particle of a substance that has all the original properties of that substance.

Monocyte—A kind of white cell that destroys bacteria and foreign particles.

Mucus—A thick fluid that protects the surfaces of the body's air passages and intestines.

Pancreas—A large gland behind the stomach that secretes pancreatic juice, which helps digest all types of food. It also secretes the hormone *insulin*, which regulates the amount of sugar in the blood.

Pancreatic juice—The most powerful and complete digestive juice, which acts on carbohydrates, fats and proteins to break them down into simpler molecules.

Papilla—A budlike structure. On the tongue, a papilla is a taste bud.

Parasympathetic nervous system—A division of the autonomic nervous system that slows the heart, aids digestion, and slows the breathing. It works against the sympathetic division, which takes over under stress to prepare the body for flight or fight.

Pituitary—A small gray gland at the base of the brain that is sometimes called the "master gland." It secretes a number of different hormones that control growth, reproduction and the rate at which the body uses energy.

Plasma—The clear, liquid part of the blood. Plasma is like lymph except that it has more protein in it. Plasma makes up three fifths of the five quarts of blood found in a normal adult body.

Platelets—Tiny oval discs found in the blood that are essential to the clotting of blood.

Pore—The tiny opening of a sweat gland in the skin.

Protein—A large group of complicated molecules chiefly made of the elements oxygen, hydrogen, carbon and nitrogen. Protein is essential for the growth and repair of living tissue.

Pulmonary artery—The artery from the right ventricle of the heart that carries oxygen-poor blood to the lungs.

Pus—The thick yellowish liquid that is the result of an infection. It contains dead white cells.

Pyloric sphincter—The circular muscle at the lower end of the stomach that controls the rate at which chyme enters the small intestine.

Red blood cells—Small, disk-shaped cells that carry oxygen in the blood. The oxygen attaches to the red pigment containing iron, called *hemoglobin*. Oxygen-rich hemoglobin is bright red. When hemoglobin is oxygen-poor, it is bluish.

Reflex—An involuntary response to particular kinds of stimulation. A reflex is rapid and requires no conscious thought. Examples: cough, sneeze, yawn, knee-jerk to a tap on the knee cap.

Scab—A crusty, dried blood clot.

Secrete—To produce a substance needed for some life process. Secretions include saliva, hormones, sweat and urine.

Serum—The noncellular fluid of the blood after all the clotting material has been removed.

Shingles—A painful rash along nerves of the trunk of the body caused by chickenpox viruses left from the childhood disease.

Shock—A condition where the circulation of the blood has been disturbed. There is less oxygen to the tissues, especially the brain. It can be caused by a number of things including injury, disease and hemorrhage.

Stimulus—Any factor that causes a living thing to react.

Stratum corneum—The topmost layer of the epithelium, containing dead, keratinized (cornified) cells.

Sweat—A watery secretion made by sweat glands and delivered to the surface of the skin. Its evaporation helps cool the body.

Sweat gland—A tiny, coiled tube that ends in a pore on the skin's surface. There are about two million sweat glands on the human body, which make about a quart of sweat a day.

Sympathetic nervous system—A division of the autonomic nervous system that acts during emergencies to prepare the body to fight or to run away.

Synapse—The point where two nerves meet and a nerve impulse passes from one nerve to another.

Thrombin—An enzyme formed during injury to a blood vessel that reacts with fibrinogen to form a blood clot.

Trachea (windpipe)—The tube that carries air from the back of the throat to the lungs. The upper end is the voice box. The lower end branches into two bronchi, which go to each lung. The trachea is held open by rings of cartilage.

Vaccine—A fluid containing weakened, dead or very diluted germs for the purpose of stimulating the body to make antibodies that will give protection against the actual disease.

Vaccination—An innoculation of a vaccine.

Vagus nerve—The main nerve of the parasympathetic nervous system, which can both carry sensations to the hypothalamus and cause reactions in organs and glands.

Vena cava—The largest vein of the body. It returns blood to the right atrium of the heart.

Villi—Tubelike extensions of cells lining the small intestine. Food is absorbed into the bloodstream by the villi.

Virus—The simplest microscopic form of life, totally dependent on other kinds of cells to eat, give off wastes and multiply. Viruses cause a variety of deseases.

Vocal bands—Two folds of tissue in the voice box that vibrate and produce a voice when air passes over them.

Voice box—The enlarged upper part of the windpipe that contains the vocal bands and is responsible for the voice. It is also called the larynx and the Adam's apple.

Warm-blooded—Describing animal life where a constant body temperature is maintained regardless of the temperature of the surroundings.

White blood cells—Blood cells that fight infection by moving to infected areas and "eating" germs. They also make antibodies to fight germs.

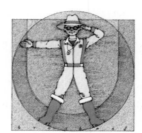

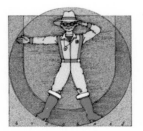

ABOUT THE AUTHOR

VICKI COBB is the renowned author of science books for young people including *Science Experiments You Can Eat, Bet You Can't! Science Impossibilities to Fool You*, and *Lots of Rot*. Her many awards include the Children's Science Book Award from the New York Academy of Science and the Eva L. Gordon Award for excellence in children's science literature.

Vicki Cobb is a graduate of Barnard College and earned a Master's degree in Secondary School Science Education from Columbia University Teachers College. She has worked as a teacher, scientific researcher, host of her own science TV show for kids, a network television newswriter, and as a publicist. Currently she spends her time writing and speaking all over the country to children, teachers, and librarians.

ABOUT THE ARTIST

JOHN SANDFORD was born in Hannibal, Missouri, and grew up in Pontiac, Illinois. As a child learning to draw, he found inspiration in a home filled with books and ideas. Mr. Sandford has illustrated numerous books of all types. He attended the American Academy of Art in Chicago, Illinois, where he works and lives with his wife, Frances.